D1215404

t

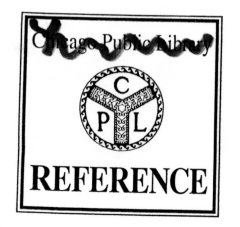

Chicago Public Library

REFERENCE

Springer
Berlin
Heidelberg
New York
Barcelona
Budapest
Hong Kong
London
Milan
Paris
Santa Clara
Singapore
Tokyo

A. Cesarani, D. Alpini, R. Boniver,
C.F. Claussen, P.M. Gagey,
L. Magnusson, L.M. Ödkvist (Eds.)

Whiplash Injuries

Diagnosis and Treatment

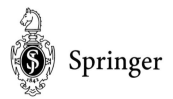

Springer

A. CESARANI
Ospedale Maggiore Policlinico, Istituto di Audiologia, Università degli Studi
di Milano, Via Sforza 35, Milan, Italy

D. ALPINI
ENT, Otoneurological Service Scientific Institute S. Maria N.te,
F.ne don Gnocchi, via Capecelatro 66 - 20148 Milan, Italy

R. BONIVER
Maître de Conférences, Université de Liège, Rue de Bruxelles 21
B-4800 Verviers, Belgium

C.F. CLAUSSEN
Neurototologic and Equilibriometry Society (NES),
Bad Kissingen, Germany

P.M. GAGEY
Institut de Posturologie, Av. de Corbera 4, Paris, France

L. MAGNUSSON
Dept of Otorhinolaryngology, University Hospital, Lund, Sweden

L.M. ÖDKVIST
Department of Otolaryngology, University Hospital,
S-58185 Linköping, Sweden

ISBN 3-540-75015-0 Springer-Verlag Berlin Heidelberg New York

© Springer-Verlag Italia, Milano 1996
Printed in Italy

Table of Contents   R0126124255

The Editors thank Pharmacia & **Upjohn** *for its support*

List of Contributors

A

Abello G. 236
Alpini D. 3, 75, 107, 206, 222, 227, 241
Ardoino P.L. 19
Atanasio S. 162

B

Barozzi S. 134
Bettinelli A. 42
Boniver R. 59, 143
Bonuccelli L. 187
Borsari C. 187
Brambilla D. 75
Brambilla S. 13, 30
Brunati L. 236

C

Casani A. 119, 187
Castello E. 149
Cesarani A. 3, 75, 107, 206, 222, 227, 241
Claussen C.F. 3

D

De Bellis M. 206
Dellepiane M. 88

E

Enock E. 200

F

Fattori B. 119, 187
Forni M. 200

X

G

Gagey P.M. 52
Garaventa G. 149
Ghilardi P.L. 119, 187

K

Karlberg M. 47

L

Leonardi M. 42
Lintura A. 200

M

Magnusson M. 47, 113
Mangiagalli E.P. 42
Mangoni A. 236
Meani E. 30
Medicina M.C. 88
Meola G. 38
Merlo E. 107
Mondini A. 13, 30
Monti B. 134

N

Negrini S. 162

O

Ödkvist I. 196
Ödkvist L.M. 64, 100, 196
Osio M. 236

P

Pallestrini E.A. 149

R

Rigo S. 82
Romanò C.L. 13, 30

S

Salami A. 88
Sansone V. 38
Savini M. 222
Sibilla P. 162
Spanio M. 82

Preface

This book is based on the proceedings and discussions of a closed workshop held in Santa Margherita Ligure in January 1995.

It was an original scientific experience: no public was admitted. For three days the main contributors of this book remained closed in a wonderful hotel. In the same hotel Guglielmo Marconi, in the 30s, performed his first experiments with radio waves. The hotel was therefore an ideal place, although the problems we discussed were not so "revolutionary" like Marconi's experiments.

In these days round tables, superrescricted meetings on specific topics and presentation of selected papers, only for very few persons, were performed. We discussed about definition, ethiopathogenesis, physiopathology, clinical and instrumental evaluations, medico-legal and therapeutic aspects of whiplash injuries.

All the attendants tried to report and discuss personal experiences and ideas in order to compare them.

All the discussions were especially aimed to prepare the chapters you will read in this book.

We returned to our homes very tired, but very rich in our minds. We really hope that after reading this book you will be as tired as rich.

We are very grateful to Pharmacia, who supported the closed workshop and the preparation of this publication.

ANTONIO CESARANI
DARIO ALPINI

PART 1

GENERAL ASPECTS

Whiplash: An Interdisciplinary Challenge

A. Cesarani, C. F. Claussen[1] and D. Alpini[2]

Definitions of whiplash syndrome are controversial. Generally speaking the syndrome comprehends symptoms following a traffic accident, usually a rear-end collision. These symptoms are varied and variably combined:
- Orthopaedic, such as neck pain and functional limitation of cervical movements
- Neurological, such as paresthesias
- Audiological, such as tinnitus and hypoacusia
- Otorhinolaryngological, such as dysphagia and disphonias
- Equilibriometric, such as vertigo and dizziness
- Odontoiatric, such as disturbances of occlusions, tempero-mandibular joint pain
- Neuropsychological, such as anxiety and attentional disturbances

The term whiplash was used for the first time in 1928 and included several mechanisms. For example the kinematics of the head-neck movements are different in rear-end collisions than in side collisions, and it is different for the driver rather than the passenger. It is also different if the subjects wore safety belts or not.

Thus the first challenge is definition. In this book whiplash injury can be defined as: A non-contact quick (< 50 ms) acceleration-deceleration head-neck trauma [13, 30, 36].

The different combinations of symptoms lead to different syndromes so described in the literature: cervical syndrome; traumatic cervical syndrome; cervico-cephalic syndrome; cervico-brachial syndrome.

Generally all syndromes are characterized by a plethora of functional symptoms and lack of sufficient objective morphological findings. Either for diagnosis or for therapy, different specialists and examinations are usually necessary; however, visit to different specialists usually leads to different "specialized" diagnosis and treatments.

Ospedale Maggiore Policlinico, Istituto di Audiologia, Università degli Studi di Milano, Via Sforza 35, Milan, Italy
[1] Neurotologic and Equilibrium Society (NES), Bad Kissingen, Germany
[2] ENT, Otoneurological Service Scientific Institute S. Maria N.te, F.ne don Gnocchi, Via Capecelatro 66, 20148 Milan, Italy

Thus the second challenge is documentation of the functional and morphological basis for the patient's complaints. Documentation is indispensable for medico-legal expertise and/or for treatment planning.

Since a patient's complaints begin with the trauma, last for months and can persist for years, the third challenge is an interdisciplinary approach to the treatment in order to avoid chronic impairment and over specialized therapy.

Whiplash injuries vary from minor to severe. They can be classified according to the Abbreviated Injury Score (Table 1). Generally the evolution of whiplash is divided into three phases:

1. The onset phase, involving local reactions with release of neuromediators such as serotonin, histamine, bradykinin and classical inflammation [7]
2. The recovery phase, locally characterized by synthesis of new collagen fibers
3. The remodelling phase, in which the neck or the body modify their positions and movement strategies in order to restore normal daily life activities

During whiplash the kinematics of the cervical spine are completely disrupted (Fig. 1). During the impact the vertebrae do not reciprocally move harmonically such as during physiological antero- and retroflexion of the neck. Whiplash is characterized by transient, but not always temporary, reciprocal inversions of the different cervical segments [60, 61, 63]. For example in the last phase of anteroflexion inversions in segments C1-C2 and C0-C1 have been observed, while in the second phase of retroflexion an inversion of the segment C0-C1 happens [64, 65]. The reciprocal inversions lead to ligament and soft tissue lesions, with a segmental disregulation causing aspecific activation of nociceptive inputs and consequent somato-motor and sympathetic-motor dysfunctions [1]. The nociceptive inputs, via interneurons and α-motoneurons, provoke a disregulation of motoneurons for the flexors and extensors leading to asymmetrical hypertonus. The latter [16-22] is generally observed in the trapezius and sternocleidomastoid with consequent compression of the accessorius nerve, and in scalenii with compression of the

Table 1. Abbreviated Injury Score (AIS)

AIS	Injury
0	No injury
1	Minor
2	Moderate
3	Serious
4	Severe
5	Critical
6	Maximum injury (virtually unsurvivable)
9	Unknown

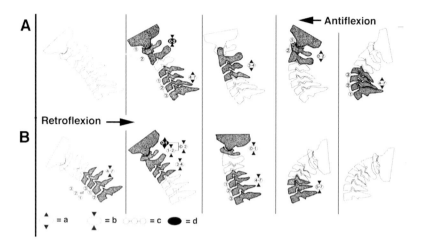

Fig. 1. Modification of reciprocal positions of cervical spine segments during anti-
(*A*) and retroflexion (*B*) in whiplash mechanisms. In the initial phase of anteroflexion
C1-2 and C0-2 invert their position *(a)*. In the second phase of retroflexion inversion
of C0-1 is observed. *a*: flexion; *b*: extension; *c*: sequence; *d*: inversion

brachial plexus, responsible for paresthesias. The dysregulation of the or-
thosympathetic cervical system causes activation of vasoconstrictive sub-
systems, not always localized to the involved segments. Vasoconstriction
induces dystrophic impairment contributing to the cervico-facial and cervico-brachial symptoms. The ganglion cervicalis superius is localized at the
C1-C4 segment and innervates the neck and extra- and intracranial upper
respiratory and digestive tracts [43].

The cervico-brachial sympathetic complex from C5 to Th1 along with the
post-ganglionate synapses in the cervical medius glangion (C5-C6) and in-
ferius (C7-C8) innervate the medium parts of the respiratory and digestive
tracts.

Cervico and cranio-spinal injuries during acceleration-deceleration lead
to head/neck proprioception disruption causing transient, sometimes permanent, abnormal proprioceptive information regarding the reciprocal position
of neck, head and trunk. In Fig. 2 the so called spino-cerebello-vestibulo-
spinal circuitry is shown. General proprioception information (from muscles, ligaments and joints) is integrated and elaborated in the cerebellum
together with special proprioception information from maculae and cristae.
From cerebellum efferent pathways return to spinal motoneurons through
another elaboration in the vestibular nuclei (with special regard to the lateral
Deiter's nucleus) [8,9, 28,29].

This circuitry is the anatomo-neurophysiological basis needed to understand why an apparent segmental injury often becomes an injury of the whole

6

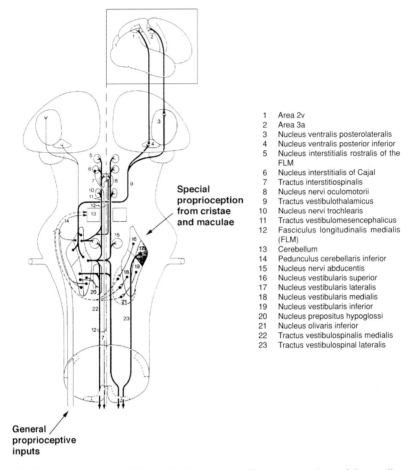

1 Area 2v
2 Area 3a
3 Nucleus ventralis posterolateralis
4 Nucleus ventralis posterior inferior
5 Nucleus interstitialis rostralis of the FLM
6 Nucleus interstitialis of Cajal
7 Tractus interstitiospinalis
8 Nucleus nervi oculomotorii
9 Tractus vestibulothalamicus
10 Nucleus nervi trochlearis
11 Tractus vestibulomesencephalicus
12 Fasciculus longitudinalis medialis (FLM)
13 Cerebellum
14 Pedunculus cerebellaris inferior
15 Nucleus nervi abducentis
16 Nucleus vestibularis superior
17 Nucleus vestibularis lateralis
18 Nucleus vestibularis medialis
19 Nucleus vestibularis inferior
20 Nucleus prepositus hypoglossi
21 Nucleus olivaris inferior
22 Tractus vestibulospinalis medialis
23 Tractus vestibulospinal lateralis

Special proprioception from cristae and maculae

General proprioceptive inputs

Fig. 2. The connections of the vestibular system: efferent connections of the vestibular nuclei and the spino-cerebello-vestibulo-spinal circuitry

individual. Equilibrium disorders can be directly caused by perturbation of integration of general with special proprioception either for abnormal peripheral inputs from the neck or for central dysfunction, particurarly of the brainstem [3, 5, 6, 14].

Whiplash is a true head trauma even if there is no contact of the head with an object. Cerebral contusions or intracranial bleeding are extremely rare but abducens mono and bilateral palsy [54] and laryngeal palsy have been described [15]. Neurovegetative symptoms and affective, cognitive symptoms are as frequent as in post-commotional syndromes and are characterized by hyperesthesic-emotional and neuroasthenic symptoms including tinnitus, dysphasia, nausea, unsteadiness, vertigo [4, 40, 42, 45, 50, 52, 62].

True neuropsychological disorders are frequent after whiplash. Typically, especially 6-8 months after the trauma, psychological symptoms appear: restlessness, nervousness, anxiety, emotional lability, difficulties in concentration, depression. In 15%-25% this neuropsychological syndrome can evolve chronically and can be misdiagnosed as an "indemnity syndrome". Experimental post-mortem studies showed focal contusions in frontal and temporal cortex, corpus callosum, subcortical structures, diencephalon and subdural and subarachnoidal microbleeding as consequences of sudden angular accelerations. Rarely alterations are macroscopic while generally, microscopic lesions have been revealed [23-25, 41, 66].

One of the central networks involved in post-whiplash disorders is the ascending reticular activating system (ARAS). Experimental studies showed involvement of the ARAS especially for translatory accelerations. In Ommaya's hypothesis [46-49] the centripetal forces during acceleration-decelaration lead to an abnormal stretching of the cerebrum with, furthermore, a sudden transient increase of the pressure of the cerebro-spinal fluid [55]. In this hypothesis whiplash provokes a commotio cerebri with potential injuries of temporal cortex, amygdala, hippocampus, medial temporal cortex, corpora mamillaria, medial thalamus, basal nuclei, prefrontal cortex, and retrosplenial cingulate cortex. All these structures may be involved in the genesis of neuropsychological symptoms [27, 30, 31].

The cerebral effects of whiplash have been studied also by Electro-Encephalography (EEG). After a period ranging from 1 to 9 years in patients with a chronic whiplash syndrome EEG alterations have been observed with percentages ranging from 30% to 49%.

Glucose cerebral metabolism has been investigated by Position Emission Tomography (PET) [26] and alterations have been shown in frontal and temporal cortex, in nucleus caudatus. Lesions of frontal cortex are responsible for attentional disorders.

The pathogenesis of otoneurological disorders is still debated and includes the following explanations:
- Mechanical compression with dynamic stenosis of the vertebral artery
- Sympathetic abnormal stimulation
- Proprioceptive disorders especially from the cervical and lumbar regions [56-58]
- Central vestibular system disorder

Probably, equilibrium disorders derive from different combinations of different mechanisms. The kinematics of the acceleration-deceleration are different, for example, for the driver, who usually opposes the trauma by means of his/her arms on the wheel, and the passenger, who usually receives, completely passively, the impact forces. Differences can be observed if patients did or did not wear safety belts duing the impact: with safety belts the movement of the head and the neck is not sagittal but torsional with the first dorsal vertebra as fulcrum. The sense of the torsional component is different: clockwise for the passenger, counterclockwise for the driver. Furthermore, rarely is the impact caused by a perfect sagittal rear-end collision, while, very often, the impact causes a rotational acceleration of the car. Torsional and angular accelerations cause microlesions in different parts of the brain, and this can lead to different combinations of signs and symptoms in the so-called whiplash syndrome [2].

Torsional and rotational acceleration-deceleration can lead to craniomandibular dysfunctions, too. Computer simulations [32] showed an initial derangement of condylus position with a myogenic secondary reaction during hyperextension and consequent modification of the condylus position. During hyperflexion the retropositioning of the condylus leads to a compression of the posterior ligament rich in vessels and proprioceptors [10, 33, 35, 51].

Following whiplash either for mechanical lesions of cervical dynamic or central dysfunctions some modifications of patient posture are usually observed [34]: the head modifies its position according to an antalgic flexion; the head reduces its rotational and latero-flexion movements. During subject movements rotation of the body is along the trunk and not the neck; the trunk is ipislaterally rotated with respect to the side of the lesion; the pelvis is rotated according to head antalgic position; the position of center of gravity (CoG) is modified. In the months following the trauma erector paravetebral muscles become hypotonic and the prevalence of flexors induces a forward displacement of the CoG facilitating forward falling. Rotation of the trunk increases unsteadiness and forward CoG displacement provokes a relative flexion of the legs to oppose falling and derangement of normal ankle and hip strategies. In fact Equitest shows a prevalence of ankle strategies and delayed motor control test latencies either in backward or in forward translations.

From a cybernetic point of view equilibrium disorders are provoked by distortion and desynchronization of the proprioceptive chain:
- Modification of the proprioceptive cervical inputs to the vestibualr nuclei and reticular formation
- Desynchronization between special vestibular inputs and general cervical inputs regarding head position and movement
- Modification of the cervico-spinal reflexes

If desynchronizations of proprioceptive signals "force" the limits of the patient's equilibrium system *calibration* (see the chapter "The Therapeutic Strategy") the system is not able to adapt and it becomes dysfunctional: vertigo and dizziness appear.

Thus the fourth challenge is correct treatment of an apparently localized injury that causes a systemic dysfunction.

The treatment must be planned on the basis of an accurate functional local and systemic diagnosis. In the acute phase treatment is aimed at reducing the impairment that is principally caused by local dysfunction. In the immediately post-acute phase impairment is due to the disregulation of somatic and vegetative reflexes at the involved spinal segment level. This disregulation, if not correctly treated, can lead to the so-called chronic phase of segmental impairment. Further evolution of the syndrome includes non-segmental disregulation: primary damage induces secondary damage. The chronic syndrome can lead to disability with motor dysfunction of the patient, usually combined with vertigo and dizziness. Rarely motor dysfunction leads to social handicap with working and/or attending to normal daily life activity no longer possible.

Rehabilitation is generally the treatment of choice either in acute or in chronic syndromes and is usually combined with drugs [59] and both physical [37-39, 44, 53] and instrumental therapies. Rehabilitation is aimed either at the treatment of the spine or at ataxia and motor uncoordination. In the chronic phase, rehabilitation must also include instruction for ergonomic daily life activities [11, 12].

Last but not least, whiplash is a medico-legal challenge. Despite the plethora of chronic symptoms, specific and pathognomonic neurological, neuropsychological and neurootological findings are usually scarce. Aspecific alterations of EEG and evoked potentials are described [31, 66]. Neurootological findings, by contrast, are more specific especially regarding posturography (static and dynamic) and each examination should not be considered *per se* but compared and integrated with the others. Thus the specificity of neurootological findings, with respect to other documentation, is not derived from one special test but from the combination of ocularmotor, vestibular, posturographic and cranio-corpographic findings.

References

1. Boquet J et al (1979) Lateralized sympathetic hyperactivity, vertigo and post-concussional syndrome after whiplash. Aggressologie 20:231-232
2. Campana BC (1988) Cervical hyperextension injuries and low back pain. In: Rosen P (ed): Emergency medicine, vol I, CV Mosby, Philadelphia, 799-817
3. Dichgans J et al (1974) The role of vestibular and neck afferents during eye-head coordination in the monkey. Brain Res 71:225-232
4. Dikmen S et al (1986) Neuropsychological and psychological consequences of minor head injury. J Neurol Neurosurg Psych 49:1227-1232
5. Doerr M et al (1984) Eye movements during active head turning with different vestibular and cervical input. Acta Otolaryngol (Stockh) 98:14-20
6. Doerr M et al (1991) Tonic cervical stimulation: does it influence eye position and eye movements in man? Acta Otolaryngol (Stockh) 111:2-9
7. Dooms GC et al (1985) Mr imaging of intramuscular bemorrhage. JCAT 9:908-913

8. Drukker J, Wal JC van der (1990) Central verbindingen van het vestibulaire apparaat. In: Fischer, AJEM, Oosterveld WJ (eds): Duizeligheid en Evenwichtsstoornissen, Data Medica, Utrecht, 29-45

9. Drukker J, Jansen JC (1975) Compendium anatomie. De Tijdstroom, Lochern

10. Eckerdahl O (1991) The petrotympanic fissure: a link connecting the tympanic cavity and the temporomandibular joint. J Craniomand Pract 9:15-21

11. Fitz-Ritson D: (1990) The chiropractic management and rehabilitation of cervical trauma. J Manipulative Physiol Ther 13:17-25

12. Foley-Nolan D et al (1990) Post whiplash dystonia well controlled by TENS: case report. J Trauma 30:909-910

13. Foreman SM, Croft AC (1988) Whiplash injuries. The cervical acceleration/deceleration syndrome. Williams & Wilkins, Baltimore

14. Gray LP (1956) Extralabyrinthine vertigo due to cervical muscle lesions. J Laryngol 70:352-361

15. Helliwell M et al (1984) Bilateral vocal cord paralysis due to whiplash indury. Br Med J 6:1876-1877

16. Hinoki M, Kurosawa T: Note on vertigo of cervical origine. Pract Otol (Kyoto) 57:10-20

17. Hinoki M (1967) Otoneurological observations on whiplash injuries with special reference to the formation of equilibrial disorder. Clin Surg (Tokyo) 22:1683-1690

18. Hinoki M (1970) Physiological role of cervical proprioceptors in the development of optic and vestibular reflexes. Adv Neurol Sci (Tokyo) 14:134-139

19. Hinoki M et al (1971) Neurotological studies on vertigo due to whiplash injury. Equilibrium Res [Suppl 1]:5-29

20. Hinoki M, Niki H (1975) Neurotological studies on the role of the sympathetic nervous system in the formation of traumatic vertigo of cervical origin. Acta Otolaryngol (Stockh) [Suppl 330]:185-196

21. Hinoki M, Ushio N (1975) Lumbomuscular proprioceptive reflexes in body equilibrium. Acta Otolaryngol (Stockh) [Suppl 330]:197-210

22. Hinoki M (1985) Vertigo due to whiplash injury: a neurotological approach. Acta Otolaryngol (Stockh) [Suppl 419]:9-29

23. Hirsch Sa et al (1988) Whiplash syndrome: fact or fiction? Orthop Clin North Am 19:791-795

24. Hodge JR (1971) The whiplash neurosis. Psychosomatics 12:245-249

25. Hodgson SP, Grundy M (1989) Whiplash injuries: their long-term prognosis and its relationship to compensation. Neuro Orthop 7:88-91

26. Humayun MS et al (1989) Local cerebral glucose abnormalities in mild closed head injured patients with cognitive impairments. Nucl Med Communic 10:335-344

27. Hofstad H, Gjerde IO (1985) Transient global amnesia after whiplash trauma. J Neurol Neurosurg Psych 48:956-957

28. Igarashi M et al (1972) Nystagmus after experimental cervical lesions. Laryngoscope 2:1609-1621

29. Ikeda K, Kobayashi T (1967) Mechanisms and origin of so-called whiplash injury. Clin Surg 22:1655-1660

30. Jenkins A et al (1986) Brain lesions detected by magnetic resonance imaging in mild and severe head injuries. The Lancet Aug 23:445-446

31. Kischka U et al (1991) Cerebral symptoms following whiplash injury. Eur Neurol 31:136-140

32. Kronn E (1990) A study on the incidence of temporomandibular dysfunction due to internal derangement in patients who have suffered from a whiplash injury. Dublin school of physiotherapy, Dublin

33. Lader E (1983) Cervical trauma as a factor in the development of TMJ dysfunction and facial pain. J Craniomand Pract 1:86-90

34. McElhaney JH et al (1976) Handbook of human tolerance. Report Japan Automobile Research Institute Inc, Yataba-Chuo, Tsukuba

35. McGlone R et al (1988) Trigeminal pain due to whiplash injury. Br J Accident Surg 19:366

36. McKenzie JA, Williams JF (1975) The effect of collision severity on the motion of the head and neck during "whiplash". J Biomech 8:257-259

37. McKinney LA (1989) Early mobilisation and outcome in acute sprains of the neck. Br Med J 299:1006-1008

38. McKinney LA et al (1989) The role of physiotherapy in the management of acute neck sprains following road traffic accidents. Arch Emerg Med 6:27-33

39. Mealy K et al (1986) Early mobilisation of acute whiplash injuries. Br Med J 292:656-657

40. Merskey K (1984) Psychiatry and the cervical sprain syndrome. Can Med Assoc 1:1119-1121

41. Miller H (1961) Accident neurosis. Br Med J 1:919-925

42. Miller Fisher C (1982) Whiplash amnesia. Neurology 32:667-668

43. Miura Y, Tanaka M (1970) Disturbances of the venous system in the head and neck regions in rabbits with whiplash injury. Brain and Nerve Injury (Tokyo) 2:217-223

44. Odent M (1975) La réflexotherapie lombaire. La Nouvelle Presse Medicale 4:26

45. Olsnes BT (1989) Neurobehavioral findings in whiplash patients with long-lasting symptoms. Acta Neurol Scand 80:584-588

46. Ommaya AK et al (1968) Whiplash and brain damage. JAMA 204:75-79

47. Ommaya AK, Gennarelli TA (1974) Cerebral concussion and traumatic unconsciousness. Brain 97:633-654

48. Ommaya AK (1985) The head: kinematics and brain injury mechanisms. The biomechanics of impact trauma. Elsevier, Amsterdam

49. Ommaya AK (1988) Mechanisms and preventive management of head injuries: a paradigm for injury control. 32nd Annual Proc of As the the Advancement of Automobile Medicine, Seattle, Sept 12-14, Washington

50. Rowe MC, Carlson C (1980) Brainstem auditory evoked potentials in post-concussion dizziness. Arch Neurol 37:670-683

51. Roydhouse RH (1973) Whiplash and temporomandibular dysfunction. Lancet 1394-1395

52. Rubin W (1973) Whiplash with vestibular involvement. Arch Otolaryngol 97:85-87

53. Seletz E (1958) Whiplash injuries: neurophysiological basis for pain and methods used for rehabilitation. JAMA 168:1750-1755

54. Shifrin LZ (1991) Bilateral abducens nerve palsy after cervical spine extension injury. Spine 16:374-375

12

55. Swenson MY et al (1990) Transient pressure changes in the spinal canal under whiplash motion. Report R-008. Dept of Injury Prevention, Chalmers University of Technology, Sweden

56. Thodem U, Mergner T (1984) Effects of proprioceptive inputs on vestibulo-ocular an vestibulospinal mechanisms. Progr in Brain Res 76:109-119

57. Ushio N et al (1971) Studies on inverted optokinetic nystagmus in cases with whiplash injury. Pract Otol (Kyoto) 64:493-509

58. Ushio N et al (1973) Studies on ataxia of lumbar origin in cases of vertigo due to whiplash injury. Agressologie 14:73-82

59. Vink R et al (1988) Treatment with the thyreotropin-releasing hormone analog CG 3703 restores magnesium homeostasis following traumatic brain injury in rats. Brain Research 460:184-188

60. White III AA, Panjabi M (1978) Clinical biomechanics of the spine. Lippincott, Philadelphia

61. Wilmink JT, Penning L (1987) Rotation of the cervical spine. A CT study in normal subjects. Spine 12:732-738

62. Winston KR (1987) Whiplash and its relationship to migraine. Headache 27:452-457

63. Wismans JSHM et al (1986) Omni-directional human head-neck response. 30 th Stapp Car Crash Conference Proceedings, San Diego, SAE paper 861893, Society of Automotive Engineers Inc, Warrendale, Usa

64. Wike BD (1967) The neurology of joints. Ann Roy Coll Surgeons Engl 41:25-50

65. Wyke BD (1979) Neurology of cervical joints. Physioter 65:72-76

66. Zomeren AH, Brouwer WH (1990) Attentional deficits after closed head injury. In: Deelman BG et al (eds): Traumatic brain injury: clinical, social and rehabilitational aspects, Swets & Zeintlinger, Amsterdam/Lisse, 33-48

Functional Anatomy

C. L. ROMANÒ, A. MONDINI AND S. BRAMBILLA

The anterior faces of the cervical column is composed by a median portion made of the overlapping of the vertebral bodies which include the intervertebral disks on top of the bodies. This median portion is at first narrowed on the top (15 mm) and is progressively broadened towards the bottom, reaching 25-30 mm at the last cervical metamer.

The superior vertebral plate of the vertebral bodies that go from C3 to C7, ends laterally with 2 osseous raized portions directed towards the top, called unciform processes or uncus. These are included with the corrisponding incisions on the lateral inferior side of the above vertebral body, functionally behaving like true articulations (Von Luschka articulations) that limit the lateral slant movement of the head.

Laterally, in corrispondence of the top half of the vertebral bodies the reliefs of the transverse processes can be noticed, and they end laterally with their anterior tuberculum. Of the latter, the C6 is called Chaissaignac's tuberculum and represents an important surgical traceable point, since it is more neatly developed in respect to the others (Fig. 1).

The intertransversal foramen are found in the middle of the transverse processes and give way to the vertebral arteries which penetrate in most cases in C6, with its veins, the vegetative nerve and the rachis nerve.

The posterior faces shows the reliefs of the spinal apophysis from C2 to C6 on the median line; and both sides of the spinal apophysis extend to 2 osseous plates that end on both sides: the first paramedian includes the series of the vertebral laminaes, lightly oblique externally, interrupted transversally by the narrow depression of the interlaminar spaces. The second lateral side is formed by the overlapping of the zygoapophysar articular processes and extends itself to the frontal plane for a median width of 15 mm.

The external border of this side is easily found because it is blunt and sticks out like a step.

A cavity separates the medial borders from the plane of the laminae: it represents an important surgical traceable point because in front of it passes the vertebral artery (Fig. 2).

Istituto Ortopedico G. Pini, Via Rugabella 4, 20122 Milan, Italy

14

Fig. 1. A Lateral view: vertebral artery *(1)* and rachis nerve *(2)* passing by the conjugate foramen. **B** Transversal section: intertransversal foramen *(4)*. Anterior tuberculum *(1)*; posterior tuberculum of the transverse process, peduncle *(3)*; spinal channel *(5)*; articular mass *(6)* with the superior articular facet *(7)*; uncus *(8)*

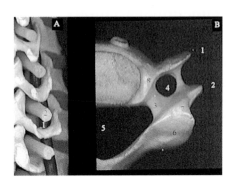

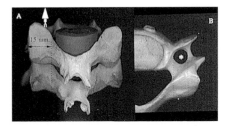

Fig. 2. A Posterior view: the articular mass has a mean width of 15 mm; a sulcus *(dotted line)*, well appreciable at surgery, separates the articular mass from the lamina; the *white arrow* shows the projection of the vertebral artery. **B** Transversal section: the *dotted line* shows the projections of the intertransversal foramen (*) on the articular mass

Viewed in the lateral projection, the cervical column shows an anterior portion formed by the alignment of the vertebral bodies, the intervertebral disks, two series of reliefs of the transverse processes and by a series of articular processes. The latter are piled on top of others to form the overall posterior articulations, characterized by an articular oblique interline, below and behind, forming an angular variation of 30°- 50° from the horizontal line. This inclination makes the superior articular process of each vertebra lie on a more anterior plane with respect to the inferior articulation of the same vertebra. The inferior articular process of a vertebra overlaps on the superior articular process of the vertebra underneath (Fig. 3).

The transverse processes are inserted in front of the articular columns via the connecting roots: an anterior one to the side of the vertebral body, and the other one posterior to the side of the articular columns, forming a cavity in front and out of the conjugate foramen through which the nerve roots abandon the rachis. The conjugate foramen is delimited superiorly and inferiorly by the peduncles in the anterior part, by the half inferior-posterior portion of the vertebral body, the lateral-posterior faces of the intervertebral disk and the unciform processes and in the posterior portion by the posterior articulation, reinforced on the anterior faces by the yellow ligament. It lies on a mildly oblique plane 20° below the horizontal plane, in front and out about 30° of the frontal plane. It has median dimensions of 12 mm in height, 6 mm in width and from 6 to 8 mm in height (Fig. 4).

These dimensions are influenced by the movements of the rachis; in fact the conjugate foramina are open during flexion, lateral angulation and rotation movements on the opposite side. They close during extention, lateral angulation and rotation movement on the same side. The horizontal or transverse section includes the vertebral cavity, anteriorly delimited by the laminae and yellow ligaments, laterally by the articular mass and by the peduncles. The vertebral foramen in the inferior cervical rachis assumes a grossly triangular form with blunted angles; the dimensions present great individual variability in the transverse and posterior diameter. The figures at both ends of anthropometric studies vary from 19 to 29 mm in the transverse sense from C3 to C7 and from 10 to 19 mm in the antero-posterior sense from C3 to C7.

The peduncles constitute osseous bridges that connect the vertebral bodies and the articular mass; their distribution is along an oblique axis directed anteriorly and medially with an angle of about 20°. On the cross section they

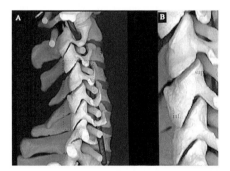

Fig. 3. Lateral view: the articular mass are superimposed to form the plane of the posterior zygoapophysar joints; their obliqueness ranges from 30°- 50° with respect to the horizontal plane

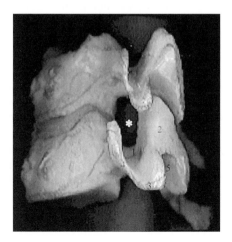

Fig. 4. Conjugate foramen (*). *(1)* peduncle; *(2)* articular mass; *(3)* transverse process; *(4)* anterior tuberculum; *(5)* posterior tuberculum

have an oval form with an axis of 10 by 7 mm. Because of the small dimensions and the tight connection close to the vertebral artery with the nerve root in the cervical rachis, the peduncles are not considered to be good joining structures, rather the articular mass is preferred.

The cervical metamers are joined together with the capsular ligament, essential for vertebral stability. The anterior longitudinal ligament is a thin ribbon-like translucent structure that without interruption extends itself on to the anterior faces of the vertebral bodies. It is intimately connected to the vertebral limitants and to the intervertebral disk, tightly adhering to the fibers of the annulus fibrosus and to a lesser degree with the central portion of the vertebral body, resulting less extent in width (Fig. 5). The annulus fibrosus appears tightly connected to the cartilage of the vertebral plates in the peripheral part, practically in continuity with the anterior and posterior longitudinal ligament. The posterior longitudinal ligament is a ribbon-like structure that extends itself along the posterior faces of the vertebral bodies, connected to the limitants and to the disk but separated from the central concave portion of the vertebral body. Its transverse extension becomes smaller from top to bottom, thereby increasing its width, which is always greater than that of anterior the longitudinal ligament (which reaches 3 mm). It limits the flexion of the rachis and the movement of the vertebral bodies, protecting the spinal cord from herniations of the discal material in a median position, while laterally leaving a breach for releasing the discal material in the connecting channel.

The articular capsules are made of dense fibrous tissue tightly attached to the osseous ends that extend horizontally for 5-7 mm. The capsular ligaments have fibers that are orthogonal faces and this allows some degree of controlled movement. When the articular faces is in the neutral position, the fibers are more relaxed. At the limit of their articular excursion the fibers are tenser, due to their orientation, limiting movement to a maximum of 3 mm with respect to the neutral position. Even the orientation of the articular faces allows flexion of the column (a controlled flexion) because it limits the outward anterior skid.

Without the articular faces, the flexion is diminished, but an outward anterior skid is seen, leading to an instability which is important to preserve in the posterior approaches of the cervical column.

The yellow ligaments represent the means of interlaminar union (Fig. 6) and are tied from half of the inner faces of the above lamina to the topmost third of the external faces of the lamina from below, and included for the most part in the vertebral channel. Normally the elasticity doesn't allow an introflexion, an impingement inside of the spinal channel during extention. Their hypertrophy, calcification or loss of elasticity due to degenerative factors can cause a dynamic stenosis with compression of the spinal marrow. The interspinous ligaments are tied between two spinal processes in an ob-

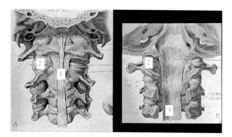

Fig. 5. A Frontal view: anterior longitudinal ligament *(1)* and zygoapophysar joints *(2)*. **B** Posterior view after removal of posterior arch: posterior longitudinal ligament *(3)*. (From [7])

Fig. 6. A Lateral view: yellow ligaments *(1)* and interspinal ligaments *(2)*. **B** Lateral view: supraspinous ligaments connect two spinal apophyses crossing each other on the median line. (From [7])

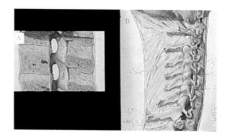

lique and posterior direction; the supraspinous ligaments are the continuation of the nucal ligaments; they connect the apex of the spinal apophysis crossing on the median line.

The cervical rachis includes nervous and vascular structures that are vitally important and, since the latter are strictly bounded to the rachis, they can be destroyed during traumatic events.

The spinal cord is in the center of the vertebral body, enveloped by three membranes (dura mater, pia mater, and arachnoid) that form the dural sac, which is suspended by the dentate ligaments, bathed in the cephalorhachidian fluid. The marrow is an elastic structure that allows itself to adapt to various movements. During extension it shortens itself and shows plicae on the surface. During flexion movements it elongates and its surface becomes smooth. The nerve roots take their origin from the spinal cord with an anterior motor branch and the sensory posterior branch. They go through a first and then a second extradural tract, starting from the opening of the conjugation channel. The posterior root forms an ovoidal swelling within the channel: the spinal ganglion. This forms an anastomosis with the anterior root, forming the spinal nerve, which divides into its two anterior and posterior branches at the exit from the conjugate channel forming the brachial plexus. The vertebral artery generally takes its origin form the subclavius artery and penetrates into C6 and goes to C1, passing through the corresponding transverse foramina. During its intrarachidial passage, it is enveloped by a sympathetic nervous plexus and by a venous plexus. Both of these structures are strictly bonded to the periosteum of the transverse foramina and are intimately attached to the nerve roots at the cross-point outside of the conjugate channel.

References

1. Callahan RA et al (1977) Cervical facet fusion for control of instability following laminectomy. J Bone Joint Surg 59A:991-1002
2. Cusick JF, Yoganandan N, Pintar F, Myklebust J, Hussain H (1988) Biomechanics of cervical spine facetectomy and fixation techniques. Spine 13:808-81
3. Halliday DR, Sullivan CR, Hollinshead WH, Bahn RC (1964) Torn cervical ligaments: necropsy examination of normal cervical region. J Trauma 4:219
4. Hollinshead WH (1965) The anatomy of the spine: points of special interest to orthopaedic surgeons. J Bone Joint Surg 47A:209
5. Kaneyama T, Hashizume Y, Ando T, Takahashi A (1994) Morphometry of the normal cadaveric cervical spinal cord. Spine 19:2077-2081
6. McLain RF (1994) Mechanoreceptor endings in human cervical facet joints. Spine 19:495-501
7. Netter FH (1978) The CIBA collection of medical illustrations. Nervous System, vol 1
8. Okada Y, Ikata T, Katoh S, Yamada H (1994) Morphologic analysis of the cervical spinal cord. dural tube, and spinal canal by magnetic resonance imaging in normal adults and patients with cervical spondylotic myelopathy. Spine 19:2331-2335
9. Panjabi MM, Pelker R, Crisco JJ, Thibodeau L, Yamamoto I (1988) Biomechanics of healing of posterior cervical spinal injuries in a canine model. Spine 13:803-807
10. Roy-Camille R (1988) Rachis cervical inferieur. Sixiemes journèes d'orthopedie de la Pitiè, Paris, Masson
11. Tominaga T, Dickman CA, Sonntag VKH, Coons S (1995) Comparative anatomy of the baboon and the human cervical spine. Spine 20:131-137
12. Vaccaro AR, Ring D, Scuderi G, Garfin S (1994) Vertebral artery location in relation to the vertebral body as determined by two-dimensional computed tomography evaluation. Spine 19:2637-2641
13. White AA, Panjiabi MM (1990) Clinical biomechanics of the spine. Philadelphia, JB Lippincott
14. Zdeblick TA, Abitbol JJ, Kunz DN, McCabe RP, Garfin S (1993) Cervical stability after sequential capsule resection. Spine 18:2005-2008
15. Zdeblick TA, Zou D, Warden KE, McCabe RP, Kunz DN, Vanderby R (1992) Cervical stability following foraminotomy: a biomechanical in-vitro analysis. J Bone Joint Surg 74A:22

Kinematics and Dynamics of the Vehicle/Seat/ Occupant System Regarding Whiplash Injuries

P. L. ARDOINO

Accident Typology at the Origin of the Whiplash

From accident analysis, it has been noticed that neck injuries are mostly caused by rear-end collisions. By way of example, we quote the following: In a Dutch study conducted in the 1980s [1], neck injuries made up 51.6% of all the lesions found in the drivers of cars involved in rear-end collisions (Table 1). In a Japanese study conducted at the beginning of the 1990s [2], the neck injury percentage in rear-end collisions increased to 80%.

A second characteristic of neck injuries is their low seriousness degree: The above-mentioned Japanese study [2] showed that, during a rear-end collision, 93% of the injuries are classified as AIS 1 level according to the Abbreviated Injury Scale [3]. As far as neck is concerned, in almost all cases, the AIS 1 level indicates a cervical rachis strain without any evidence of anatomical lesions. The same trend is emphasized in a recent study conducted in Germany [4] on a sample of about 10500 car collisions.

With regard to the rear-end collision typology, in the above-mentioned German study [4], center and off-set crashes make up about 73% of all the rear-end collisions (Fig. 1); only 27% present an angled direction.

It is necessary to point out that in low impact speed off-set crashes the off-centering does not produce notable rotations in the hit vehicle, as is regularly noticed in damageability tests with off-center crashing barriers and above 20 km/h crash speeds.

On the basis of what has been said above, we can conclude that, in almost all cases, whiplash injuries happen in a low impact speed, rear-end collision in which the speed variation takes place on the longitudinal axis of the vehicle.

Whiplash Injury Mechanism

In a rear-end collision, the chest is pushed forwards by the seatback; the burden on the neck results from the strength of inertia that works through the

FIAT Auto SpA, Direzione Tecnica, Coord. Tecn./Leg. Sicurezza, Orbassano (TO)

Table 1. Distribution of injuries by body region for several collision types, driver only [1]

	Main group	Lateral collisions	Front to front	Rear collisions	Total (including other types)
1	Skull and brain	23.7	20.0	14.4	22.2
2	Face	11.2	21.1	7.2	16.1
3	Neck	4.4	3.7	51.6	6.9
4	Thorax	20.2	16.9	6.8	16.5
5	Abdomen	2.6	2.3	0.4	2.3
6	Back	2.4	1.3	4.0	2.4
7	Pelvis	5.0	1.3	0.4	2.0
8	Arms	16.0	13.6	7.2	14.2
9	Legs	14.5	19.8	6.0	17.3
	Total	100%	100%	100%	100%

center of gravity of the head in a front-back direction; in this case, the neck injury mechanism is one of hyperextension and tension ("traction" in mechanical terminology) of the cervical rachis (Fig. 2). It should be pointed out that not all hyperextension/tension injury mechanisms are caused by whiplash.

Technical and Structural Limits

The technical norms now in force in Europe prescribe that the seatback must be able to withstand the application of a static moment of 53 (m.daN).

Even though from a theoretical point of view it is not possible to define a dynamic stress that is equivalent to the static one, on the basis of experimental data and for normal seats with 50% male anthropometric characteristics, we can consider that such a burden corresponds to the capacity to withstand the chest's inertia load in a rear-end collision between vehicles of equal mass with a closure speed of about 35 km/h.

Ignoring the retaining action of the headrest, we can deduce that for speed variations of the vehicle higher than 18 km/h the seatback can rotate backwards absorbing part of the chest kinetic energy; this phenomenon in fact limits both the angle of rotation of the head and the value of the extension moment.

The technical norms assure that the headrest withstands additional loadings compared to the seatback.

We can therefore conclude that the crash that must be considered is a rear-end one at $\Delta V < 18$ km/h with a longitudinal movement of the passenger compartment.

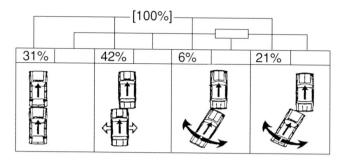

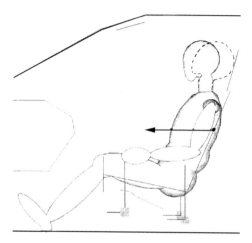

Fig. 1. Distribution of the rear accidents with injured occupants by impact type [4]

Fig. 2. Injury mechanism in whiplash

Phases of the Collision

We can identify three different phases in a rear-end collision:
- First phase: crash between the vehicles until the struck one assumes the speed variation (ΔV) due to the impact conditions
- Second phase: interaction between the seat and its occupant
- Third phase: loadings on the occupant

The three phases surely are linked and, temporarily, partially overlapping.

First Phase

Regardless of the initial speed of the two vehicles, the struck one in this phase assumes a speed variation that is a function of the masses of the vehicles, their closure speed and the spring restitution coefficient: the analytic expression of the speed variation of the vehicle that is hit is the following:

$$\Delta VA = \frac{MA \times MB}{MA + MB} (VA - VB)(1 + e)$$

where:

A	=	struck vehicle
B	=	striking vehicle
V	=	speed at the impact
ΔV	=	speed variation
M	=	mass
e	=	spring restitution coefficient
(VA - VB)	=	closure speed

The higher or lower stiffness of the vehicles brings a different degree of deformation and therefore influences the duration of the collision and the values of average acceleration, but does not modify the extent of the variation in speed.

Second Phase

The variations in motion of the hit vehicle are also those of the fastening of the seat to the body shell; the seat, mostly the seatback, is the element through which the occupant adapts its motion situation to the final one of the hit vehicle.

In a rear impact, the seatback is the actual restraint system of the occupant, just as the seatbelt is in a frontal impact.

It is important to point out that the fact of wearing the seatbelt does not influence the kinematics and the dynamics of the occupant during a lengthwise rear-end collision; the only function of the seatbelt in this particular case is to hold the occupant once the crash is over.

Two characteristics of the seat influence the stress transfer from the vehicle to the occupant: (1) the seat foam which cushions the stresses, filters and further offsets the small transversal and rotational movements of the vehicle; (2) the elasticity of the seatback structure which obviously acts only in situations which do not exceed the structural limits indicated before.

The relative head/headrest position plays a basic role in the extension/traction movement of the neck and therefore in limiting the whiplash injuries.

Third Phase

The human body is an articulated system of body segments which are submitted to external loads, applied mainly through the seat, and that interact
among themselves. In order to analyse the stresses on the single body segments, an experimental rear-end collision test has been carried out on a crash
simulator with the previously described conditions (Fig. 3).

A 17 km/h variation in speed has been applied to the passenger compart-
ement with an acceleration curve corresponding to a rear-end collision with
a rigid moving barrier and, therefore, a particulary severe one (Fig. 4).

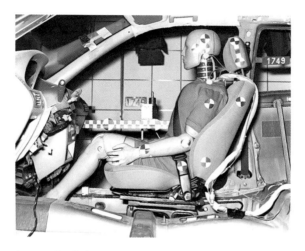

Fig. 3. Rear impact simulation. Test configuration

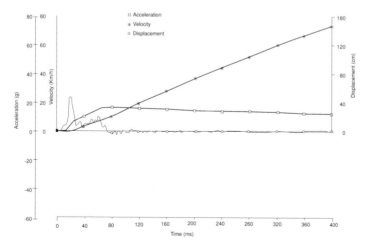

Fig. 4. Time histories of the passenger compartment

A Hybrid III dummy has been used in the front passenger position, provided with the necessary instrumentation in order to obtain (Fig. 5): (1) the pelvis, chest and head accelerations; (2) the axial loads (compression and traction), the moments (flection and extension) and the shear force on the neck; (3) the rotation of the head with regard to the basis of the neck.

Figure 6 shows the time histories (acceleration, velocity, displacement) of the occupant's pelvis, chest and head in the direction of the applied forces that, in this particular case, were horizontal-longitudinal.

It is necessary to point out that the head's speed and displacement values above 130 ms do not correspond to the actual values of the speed and displacement components along the X axis, due to the rotation of the head.

It is therefore evident that the stresses on the three body segments have different values and are transmitted in different times.

The pelvis compared with the chest is subject to a stress that is shorter lasting, with an average acceleration value which is higher, but which has a variation in speed which does not exceed that of the vehicle (17 km/h); this means that, at pelvis level, the seat and the seatback cushion the crash and do not elastically return energy to the pelvis itself.

The duration of the stress on the chest is longer due to the spring restitution of the seatback which, with a coefficient of about a 0.3, brings the chest's variation in speed to about 23 km/h.

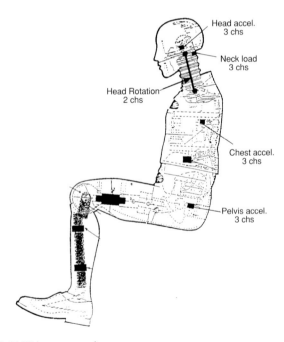

Fig. 5. Hybrid III instrumentation

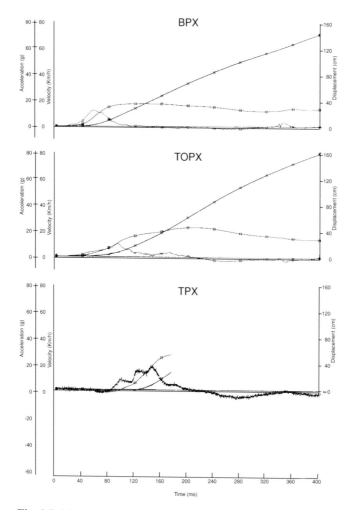

Fig. 6. Pelvis, chest, head time histories. X: horizontal longitudinal direction; P: front passenger; B: pelvis; TO: chest; T: head

Regarding the head, though we do not have the exact value of the variation in speed along the horizontal longitudinal axis, we have noticed a higher stress degree both in terms of mean acceleration and variation in speed.

The head's increase in speed variation compared to that of the chest is mainly due to the neck's spring restitution.

It should be noted that all the recorded acceleration values are at least one order of magnitude below the human tolerance levels universally accepted in the biomechanic field for these body segments.

The fact, which is also emphasized by the accident analysis, that in rear-end collisions of this severity no pelvis, chest or head injuries occur, does not alter the significance of the dynamic and kinematic trends of the system which are the input conditions for the analysis of stresses on the neck.

The overlapping of the pelvis and chest speed curves (Fig. 7) shows how, in the time interval between 80 and 200 ms, the variation in speed between chest and pelvis passes from about -10 to +7 km/h.

The same behaviour has been noticed between head and chest (Fig. 8).

Regarding stresses on the neck (moments and axial loads) (Fig. 9), we noticed a time correspondence with the acceleration of the head; the same can be said for the rotation of the head with regard to the basis of the neck.

The head acceleration and speed curves (Fig. 6) show, at about 80 ms, a small backward movement of the head, due to the lever effect of the pelvis, chest and seatback, to which a small bending moment value corresponds (Fig. 9).

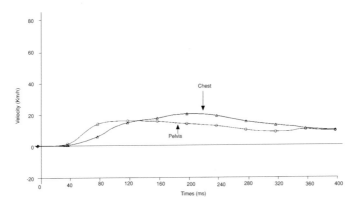

Fig. 7. Pelvis, chest velocity vs time

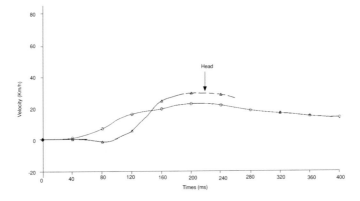

Fig. 8. Chest, head velocity vs time

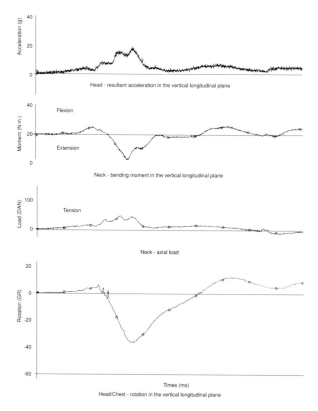

Fig. 9. Head and neck loadings

By examining Figs. 6 and 9, the following can be noted:
- The chest starts its forward movement, pushed by the seatback, at about 50 ms.
- The rotation of the head starts at about 90 ms.
- The head's center of gravity starts to shift forwards at about 120 ms.
- The maximum stresses on head and neck occur at about 150 ms.

Based on what was mentioned above, it is clear that the neck - the link between chest and head - is stressed in different ways during the crash (Fig. 10):

1. Between 50 and 90 ms the chest moves forwards and the head stays in its rest position; the neck is essentially subject to small shear strains.
2. Between 90 and 120 ms the forward movement of the chest continues; the head rotates due to the fact that the neck is subject to the application of an extension moment.
3. Between 120 and 150 ms the head continues to turn and also moves forwards pulled by the neck and pushed by the headrest. In this phase the

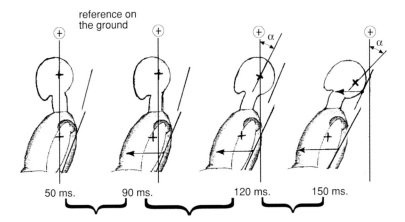

Fig. 10. Neck loadings and kinematics

neck is subject to the largest stress of extension moment and traction force and whiplash injuries occur.

Notice how, up to 200 ms (Fig. 6), and therefore after the largest stresses on the neck have taken place, the occupant is in contact with and is meanwhile pushed by the seatback; the seatbelt up to now has not exercised any restraining action and can not therefore alter in any way the kinematics and dynamics of the occupant.

Angled Rear-End Collisions

Regardless of the kind of rear-end collision, it is the seat which induces the stresses on the occupant. In the case of mainly centered angled rear-end collisions (Fig. 11), which means angles not larger than 15°- 20°, the seat moves towards the occupant along the collision direction and the stress components along the longitudinal axis represent about 95% of the total stress.

The neck injury mechanism is always an extension and tension one. In the worst case, the movement occurs on a vertical plane tilted about 15°- 20° with regard to the vertical longitudinal plane. In this case, due to the small size of the angle, the human tolerance values in terms of extension moment and traction force could slightly differ from those universally accepted in the biomechanic field for longitudinal loads.

In the remaining kinds of off-set angled rear-end collisions, the rotation of the hit vehicle dominates; the vehicle/occupant interaction does not take place solely through the seat, and therefore the whiplash stress on the neck is unlikely to occur.

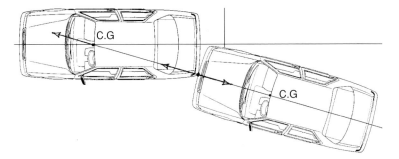

Fig. 11. Centered angled rear collision; *CG*, center of gravity

Out of Position Whiplash

Particular attention should be paid to the whiplash that occurs when the occupant is out of position; for example, just think what the neck injury mechanism could be if the stresses described above were applied to a head that initially is rotated around its vertical axis of about 60°.

Very little knowledge is available on the human tolerance and on the biomechanics of the rotated neck in the rear impact; nevertheless an injured out of position occupant should show an asymmetric lesion or symptomatology.

The necks of the current dummies do not allow us to study the injuries that could result in these situations of asymmetric and compound stresses; in fact, their biofidelity is limited to the longitudinal-vertical plane and the neck structure is symmetric with regard to any plane that passes through its vertical axis.

References

1. Van Kampem LTB Hoofdsteunen in personenauto's. Institute for Road Safety Research, SWOV, The Netherlands
2. Koshiro Ono (1993) Influences of the physical parameters on the risk to neck injuries in low impact speed rear-end collisions. Proceedings of IRCOBI, Conference
3. The Abbreviated Injury Scale (1990) Revision Association for the Advancement of Automotive Medicine (USA)
4. Verband HUK (1994) Fahrzeugsicherheit 90. Munchen

Whiplash Lesions: Orthopaedic Considerations

E. Meani, S. Brambilla, A. Mondini and C. L. Romanò

Introduction

The term whiplash was introduced for the first time by Crowe, in 1928, during a meeting of the Western Orthopaedic Association. Later, it was Davis, in 1945, who used this term in a publication about traumatic lesions of the cervical column.

Whiplash usually stands for a syndrome characterized by a soft tissue lesion of the neck (muscles, ligaments, capsules, intervertebral disk, spinal marrow, nerve roots, veins and arteries, sympathetic system).

Normally though, this term is used in a broader way to define the majority of traumatic events that involve the cervical rachis following street accidents. In this context whiplash doesn't represent a clinical syndrome, but rather comprises a group of pathological entities that are extremely different in their entity, prognosis and treatment.

Clinical Course

In an acute phase right after the trauma, the symptomatology is characterized by pain in the cervical and occipital areas, with the addition of the scapular girdle and the dorsal region; the tendency is to reach a peak in the following hours and days with establishment of a muscular contracture of the paravertebral muscles (trapezius muscle and the long muscles of the back).

These symptoms are totally aspecific and are mostly all present in the traumatic affections of the rachis; there is no relationship between the extent of the symptomatology and the gravity of the lesions.

Normally, in the acute phase, no signs of involvement of the myeloradicular structures of the rachis are present. If these signs were evident, they indicate a lesion of the soft tissues and the osteoarticular structures.

The symptomatic pain can completely resolve itself in a variable period of time from the traumatic event, or it can become chronic. The clinical

Istituto Ortopedico G. Pini, Via Rugabella 4, 20122 Milan, Italy

course is worsened with symptoms such as headache, nausea, tinnitus, lack of concentration, photophobia, retroorbital pain, anxiety, depression, easy irritability, sleep disturbances, dysesthesias of the upper limbs.

Neck pain is determined by contracture of the paravertebral cervical muscles and is accompanied by a limitation of the articular excursion; the most involved muscles (sternocleidomastoid, scalene, trapezius, long neck muscles) can determine lesions that go from simple stretching to rupture with the formation of intrafascicular hematomas. The same stretching lesions can also involve the anterior and posterior long ligaments.

Less frequent are cleavages and lacerations of the annulus fibrosus, separation of the somatic limiting of the cartilagenous plate, and lesions that can predispose to discal degeneration, which contributes to prolonging the symptomatic pain.

With some frequency, pain in the interscapular and high dorsal regions has been reported, expression of the myofascial lesions of the trapezius, rhomboid, levator of the scapular muscles, and large dentate muscle.

If the brachial pain and paresthesias are not tied to an irritative-compressive factor of the nerve roots (discal protrusion, stenosis of the conjugate channel, compression of a fractured articular apophysis) they do not generally present with a precise metameric distribution and remain difficult to interpret, even if they have been indicated as a possible cause of lesions associated with the brachial plexus or with a thoracic outlet syndrome.

Headache in the occipital area is a common symptom; generally it is due to a painful muscular spasm of the semispinal muscles and rectus muscles of the head and neck, or splenius muscle, or to stretching or laceration of the nucal ligaments. Often, in association, there is a neuralgia of Arnold's large occipital nerve.

The retroorbital pain and the reading fatigue that are often included in the complaints of patients with whiplash injuries could be tied to a proprioception problem of the paravertebral muscles, with major involvement of the intrinsic oculomotor system.

The primary lesions of the labyrinthic structures, occuring right after the trauma, would be the basis of the vertigo and would lead to incorrect posture control, the latter responsible for the abnormal state of contracture of the neck muscles.

Diagnosis

Considering the aspecificity of the clinical picture we think it is necessary to recur to a radiographic examination in a patient suffering from traumatic injury of the spine. It should include, apart from the classical frontal and lateral projections, the oblique and transoral projections, all easily performable exams in an emergency room. Fundamentally important is good execution and interpretation of the above exams: the lateral projection assesses alignment of the vertebral bodies (anterior and posterior somatic lines), the normal orientation of the articular faces and the absence of fanning of the spinal apophysis.

The anterior-posterior projection is used to evaluate the correct alignment of the spinal apophysis, the peduncles and the normal position of the vertebral bodies and the articular mass (Fig. 1).

In case of abnormal position of the vertebrae in these two standard projections, it is good to recur to the oblique projections, especially in cases that too often are thought to be partial dislocations. The oblique projections can better point out the posterior articular structures and the peduncles and better appreciate the normal conformation and dimension of the conjugate foramina (Fig. 2).

Furthermore, it is necessary to remember that, at the moment of the trauma, an extensive anthalgic muscular contraction can hide a grave lesion of the capsular, disk, ligament structures (severe sprain). However, this will eventually become clear with execution of radiographs in the lateral projection in maximal flexion and extention positions.

Dynamic radiographs will evaluate signs of vertebral instability that consist of: (1) anterolisthesis of a vertebral body with respect to the one underneath and > 3 mm; (2) loss of contact and alignment of the zygoapophysial articular surfaces > 50%; (3) increase of the interspinal distance with respect to the upper or lower metamers (fanning); (4) elective discal kyphosis; (5) angulation of the posterior somatic wall ≥ 15° (Fig. 3).

The simultaneous presence of at least three of the above radiographic signs suggests a severe sprain, an instable lesion that implies a surgical type of treatment.

A partial dislocation or a lesion that in the lateral projection points out a mild anterior sliding of a vertebral body with respect to the one underneath cannot be underestimated, because it is often tied to an unilateral lesion (fracture or dislocation of a articular apophysis, pillar fracture); the rotation type implies a mild skid in an antero-posterior sense. In this case, even if the standard projection can point out a correct diagnosis (loss of an alignment of

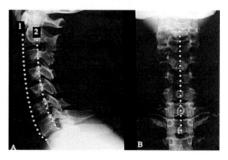

Fig. 1. A Lateral view: anterior somatic line *(1)*; posterior somatic line *(2)*. **B** The *dotted line* shows the correct alignment of the spinal apophyses

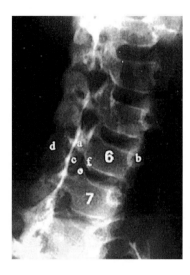

Fig. 2. Oblique view: *(a)* peduncle of C6; *(b)* peduncle of C6 from the contralateral side; *(c)* intratransversal foramen; *(d)* articular mass; *(e)* C7 uncus; *(f)* semilunar facet

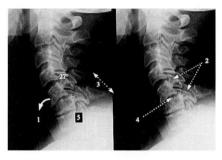

Fig. 3. Severe whiplash trauma; radiographic signs of instability. See text for explanation

the spinal apophysis in the frontal projection; doubling of the articular apophysis silhouette in the lateral projection), the oblique projections eliminate all doubts and indicate correct treatment (Fig. 4).

In the unilateral fractures, there is an eventual decomposition of the articular apophysis and its rime (frequently the top ones) or, in case of dislocation, there is a stenosis in the conjugate foramina and loss of the normal alignment of the zygoapophysial articular surfaces (Fig. 5).

In the pillar fracture of the facial mass, the characteristic sign is the horizontalization of the articular mass. This happens because this peculiar cervical rachis lesion is characterized by two rimes of fracture: the anterior one in the peduncle and the posterior one within the laminae that isolate the articular mass, which is completely torn off and can rotate downward and forward losing its normal oblique position in the lateral projection (Fig. 6).

The CT scan in this case will better evidence the two rimes of fracture, while in unilateral lesions it will confirm the diagnosis and show other lesions such as lamina fractures, not well distinguished with traditional radiology (Fig. 7). The coming of new imaging techniques, especially MRI has allowed demonstration of lesions which could previously not be pointed out. These are: rupture of the anterior longitudinal ligament, osteochondral detachments of the vertebral plate, cleavages of the annulus fibrosus, separation of the intervertebral disk from the vertebral plate, discal protrusion, the latter frequently found.

The high cost of this exam highly limits its use, now reserved for patients who show persisting algesic symptomatology with radiation to the upper limb and with paresthesias, even if the metameric distribution is not precise.

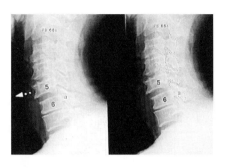

Fig. 4. In the lateral view the articular mass are usually shown as one image as the articular apophyses are superimposed on each other. In this case of unilateral fracture-dislocation of C6, the articular mass present a double profile due to the rotational component. The *arrow* shows the mild shift typical for unilateral lesions

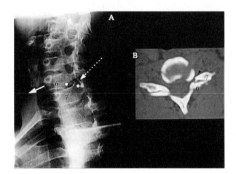

Fig. 5. A Unilateral fracture-dislocation C6-C7. The *arrow* shows the absence of normal alignment of zygoapophysial articular surfaces. The *asterisks* show the altered relationship between uncus and the semilunar facet. **B** The CT scan points out the stenosis of the conjugate channel *(arrow)*

Fig. 6. Fracture of the articular mass of C5. **A** Lateral view, showing a mild sliding of C5 over C6. **B** Oblique view: the articular mass of C5 *(*)* is anteriorly and downward rotated, narrowing the conjugate foramen of C4-C5

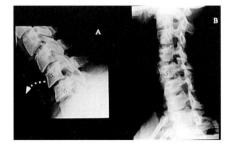

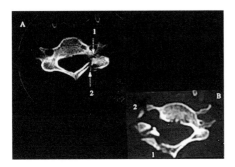

Fig. 7. A Fracture of the articular mass. The CT scan shows the fracture of the peduncle *(1)* and a second fracture line at the junction between the lamina and the articular mass *(2).* **B** In unilateral lesions the CT scan can show associated lesions, like fracture of the lamina *(1)* and *(2)* of the transverse process

Treatment

The initial phase of treatment of mild distortional foms of whiplash involves immobilization with a rigid or Phyladelphia type collar for a period of time not less than 2 weeks.

From a pharmacological point of view, the patient will benefit from the administration of analgesics (NSAIDs), myorelaxants (more efficient if with central action) and antivertigo drugs. With the removal of the orthopaedic support, it will be important to restore muscular tone to guarantee correct posture and kinematics of the cervical column: this is possible with physical training and stretching.

It is useful to combine gymnastics with physiokinetic therapy, massage therapy, TENS, and ultrasound, which all have analgesic action. Vertebral manipulation is still controversial, particularly in elderly subjects in whom degenerative alterations of the cervical rachis are present, due to the risk of permanent neurologic lesions.

In a later phase, the persisting algesic symptomatology in some patients can be relieved by the infiltration of steroid compounds in the posterior articular facies, possibly associated with local anesthetics.

Noninvasive treatment is normally undertaken in the true forms of whiplash or in mild traumatic sprain (mentioned earlier). This includes most of the traumatic events occurring in the cervical column and, as mentioned above, can lead to loss of rachis stability for osteo, disk, capsular, and ligament lesions, immediately or after the initial trauma. Instability, meaning the loss of the normal vertebral structure, needs more substantial treatment, such as more extreme immobilization with, e.g. the Halo-Vest for lesions in which the instability is exclusively or almost all osseous (thus temporaneous), with the possibility of treatment by consolidation of the fracture (pillar fracture without radicular lesion).

Surgical treatment is suggested for permanent instable forms (severe sprain, decomposition articular fractures, unilateral dislocations, pillar fracture with severe decomposition and simultaneous radicular lesion) and with protusions, discal hernias with medullar radicular lesion.

The surgical options include intersomatic diskectomy, arthrodesis performed anteriorly by Smith and Robinson's technique, possibly associated with a plaque screwed on to the upper and lower vertebral bodies, and posterior osteosynthesis by screwing together the articular mass, perhaps associated with arthrodesis (Figs. 8 and 9).

Forensic Medicine Considerations

Standard negative radiographs cannot always exclude articular lesions (from bone or from ligament) that preclude cervical articular instability.

There is not always an association between the CT and/or MRI reports (cervical discal hernias) and the clinical picture. A lot of discal diseases are preexisting to the trauma, more often in patients older than 30-35 years (inferior cervical arthritis, etc.).

The psychological aspect can't be undervalued (sometimes a real erethism of the patient) (anxious contractural affective syndrome → dorsal rachis study).

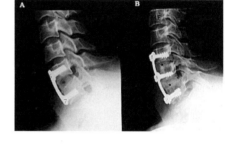

Fig. 8. Intersomatic arthrodesis performed by an anterior approach: at one level (**A**) or two levels (**B**) with different osteosynthesis devices. *Asterisks* indicate the autologous bone graft

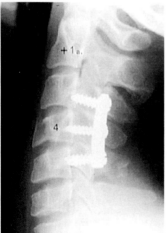

Fig. 9. Osteosynthesis with plate of the articular mass via a posterior approach

Recent retrospective studies have demonstrated that, after a 10 year period, in none of the 40 cases studied, there were subjective and objective symptoms of an earlier violent cervical sprain (earlier defined as severe sprains and therefore subject to indemnity).

References

1. Beyer CA, Cabanela ME, Berquist TH (1991) Unilateral facet dislocations and fracture-dislocations of the cervical spine. J Bone Joint Surg 73B:977-981
2. Bohlman HH (1979) Acute fractures and dislocations of the cervical spine. J Bone Joint Surg 61A:1119-1141
3. Braakman R, Vinken PJ (1967) Unilateral facet interlocking in the lower cervical spine. J Bone Joint Surg 49B:249-257
4. Clark CR, Igram CM, El-Khoury GY, Ehara S (1988) Radiographic evaluation of cervical spine injuries. Spine 13:742-747
5. Davis SJ, Teresi LM, Bradley WG, Ziemba MA, Bloze AE (1991) Cervical spine hyperextension injuries: MR findings. Radiology 180:245
6. Dosch JC, Dupuis M (1986) Le syndrome de l'antélisthésis cervical lateralisé. Radiologie J CEPUR 6:151-156
7. Dvorak J, Froelich D, Penning L, Baumgartner H, Panjabi MM (1988) Functional radiographic diagnosis of the cervical spine: flexion/extension. Spine 13:748-755
8. Evans D (1976) Anterior cervical subluxation. J Bone Joint Surg 58B:318-321
9. Fuentes JM, Benezech J, Lussiez B, Vlahovitch B (1986) La fracture-separation du massif articulaire du rachis cervical inferieure. Ses rapports avec la fracture-dislocation en hyperextension. Rev Chir Orthop 72:435-440
10. Louis R (1977) L'instabilitè. Les theories de l'instabilitè. Rev Chir Orthop 63:423
11. Roy-Camille R (1988) Rachis cervical inferieur. Sixiemes journèes d'orthopedie de la Pitiè, Paris, Masson
12. White AA, Panjiabi MM (1990) Clinical biomechanics of the spine. Philadelphia, JB Lippincott

The Neurological Point of View

G. Meola and V. Sansone

Whiplash refers to the sudden hyperextension followed by flexion of the neck that occurs when an occupant of a motor vehicle is hit from behind by another vehicle. This is such a typical mode of action determining pain in the neck that this same term is known in other languages as well: in Italian it is known as "colpo di frusta", in French it is known as *"le coup de lapein"* and in German as *"schleudertrauma"*.

The whiplash mechanism of injury is believed to be due by many clinicians to a myofascial injury. Both animal and human studies have demonstrated structural damage from whiplash type injuries ranging from muscle tears, rupture of anterior longitudinal and other ligaments to disc herniations, and retropharyngeal hematomas, depending on the forces intervening in the collision [1, 3, 4].

From an epidemiological point of view, rear-end collisions are responsible for about 85% of all whiplash injuries [1]. Women are more susceptible than men to whiplash injuries. The greater susceptibillity of women to whiplash injuries might be due to a narrower neck and a smaller muscular mass in women.

Clinical Presentation

From a clinical point of view symptoms and signs resulting from whiplash injuries vary from more commom symptoms, like neck and back pain, to headaches, dizziness and paresthesias, to more rarely complained of symptoms [2] including visual symptoms, torticollis, transient global amnesia, etc. (see Tables 1-2).

The first point which is worth emphasizing is that a significant minority of neurologists question the existence of persistent symptoms and some tend to question the authenticity of patients' reports of symptoms.

Dipartimento di Neurologia and I Divisione di Neurologia, Università di Milano, Ospedale Clinicizzato - 20097 San Donato Milanese (MI), Tel. (39)-2-52774480, Fax (39)-2-5274717, Italy

Table 1. Frequent complaints of whiplash injury

Neck and back pain	within 6 hours: 65%
	24 hours: 28%
	72 hours: 7%
Headaches	• muscle tensive type
	• greater occipital neuralgia
	• temporo-mandibular joint associated pain
	• migraine
Dizziness	• vertigo: 50%
	• floating sensation: 35%
	• tinnitus: 14%
	• hearing impairment: 5%
Paresthesias	• brachial plexopathy
	• cervical radiculopathy
Weakness	• brachial plexopathy
	• cervical radiculopathy
Cognitive disturbances	• memory defects, attentivness impairment
associated with	• irritability, nervousness
whiplash injury	• fatiguability
	• sleep disturbances
	• personality changes
Visual defects	• convergence defects
associated with	• impairment of pursuit or saccadic movement
whiplash injury	• Horner syndrome
	• oculomotor palsy

Table 2. Rare symptoms associated with whiplash injury

Torticollis
Transient global amnesia
Hypoglossal nerve palsy
Laryngeal nerve palsy

The second point is that often patients, although authentically affected, complain of symptoms which they "feel" and which prove to be not objectively demonstrable with standard procedures. This does not mean the patient is reporting nonexisting symptoms but rather that the psychological substrate of the individual and the way whiplash has affected his everyday life should be considered more deeply.

Over 60% of patients presenting to the emergency room after a motor vehicle accident complain of neck pain. The onset of back pain occurs within 6 hours in 65% of patients, within 24 hours in the additional 28% and within 72 hours in the remaining patients. Most neck pain is due to a cervical sprain or a myofascial injury [5].

Over 80% of patients complain of headaches that are occipitally located in 46% of patients, generalized in 34% and in other locations in 20%. The pain was present more than half the time in 50% of patients and was usually due to muscle contraction. Occasionally whiplash injuries can precipitate recurring common, classic and basilar migraines.

Approximately 50% of patients complain of vertigo, 35% of floating sensations, 14% of tinnitus and 5% of hearing impairment. Post-traumatic dysfunction of the vestibular apparatus, brainstem, cervical sympathetics, verterbal insufficiency and cervical proprioceptive system have all been postulated as causing dizziness.

Around 30% of patients complain of paresthesias immediately after injury without objective findings and around 37% report paresthesias after around 20 months. Paresthesias can be referred from trigger points, brachial plexopathy, cervical radiculopathy and spinal cord compression.

Cognitive and psychological symptoms usually occur in patients with chronic symptoms of whiplash injury and they include nervousness and irritability in 67%, cognitive disturbances in 50%, sleep disturbances in 44%, fatiguability in 40%, disturbances of vision in 37%, symptoms of depression in 37%. In fact most neurologists believe that prolonged symptoms are psychogenic in origin and over 18% believe that emotional factors are most responsible for whiplash symptoms. Thus psychologic factors such as neurosis are commonly cited as the cause of persistent symptoms [7].

Radiographic Findings

This is an important issue in that it is often difficult to establish what is new and what findings are pre-existing after whiplash injury: cervical spondylosis and degenerative disc disease occur with increasing frequency with older age and are often asymptomatic.

Prognosis

Because of the many symptoms and different emotional reactions to whiplash injury, it is often difficult to determine precise prognostic factors. Studies on the prognosis are difficult to compare because of multiple methodological differences, including selection criteria for patients, duration of follow-up and treatments used [6]. Multiple studies have documented that neck pain and headaches persist in significant numbers of patients: neck pain was present after 1 year in 26% of patients and was still present in 29% of patients after 2 years. Headaches are present after 1 month in 80% of patients, in over 70% after 3 months and last after 10 years in over 30% of patients.

The following *risk factors* have been reported for persistent symptoms: older age, pre-existing back pain or paresthesias, pre-existing degenerative osteoarthritic changes, cervical stenosis and abnormal cervical spine curves. A positive neurological examination is also a negative prognostic factor.

Many clinicians believe that persistent symptoms are often due to pending litigation in the medico-legal system. These symptoms promptly resolve once the litigation is completed. However the clinician should not support bias against patients just because they have pending litigations. The clinician should evaluate each case individually and learn to identify patients who exaggerate their symptoms or lie about persistent complaints to help or make their legal case.

In conclusion this paper briefly covers the epidemiology, pathology, symptoms and signs and prognosis of whiplash injuries; it is worthwhile to emphasize that, besides a neurological documentation, the physician should adopt a multidisciplinary approach in the evaluation of each case individually.

References

1. Deans GT, McGailliard JN, Rutherford WH (1986) Incidence and duration of neck pain among patients injured in car accidents. Br Med J 292:94-95
2. Dukes IK, Bannerjee SK (1993) Hypoglossal nerve palsy following hyperextension neck injury. Injury 24:133-134
3. Evans RW (1992) Some observations on whiplash injuries. Neurol Clin 10:975-977
4. Evans RW, Evans RI, Sharp MJ (1994) The physician survey on the post-concussion and whiplash syndromes. Headache
5. Kellgren JH. (1938) A preliminary account of referred pain arising from muscle. Br Med J 1:325-327
6. Norris SH, Watt I (1993) The prognosis of neck injuries resulting from rear-end vehicle collision. J Bone Joint Surg 65B:608-611
7. Radanov BP, Di Stefano G, Schnidrig A et al. (1993) Cognitive functioning after common whiplash: a controlled follow-up study. Arch Neurol 50:87-91

The Radiological Evaluation

A. BETTINELLI, M. LEONARDI AND E. P. MANGIAGALLI

The term "whiplash syndrome" was introduced by Crowe in 1928 [1] and it is normally used to describe a group of symptoms variously associated and with unequal clinical importance.

In most instances the symptomatology is subjective, therefore the ensuing radiological evaluation may be elusive.

Generally speaking, patients complain about continuous pain to the posterior aspect of the occiput or the neck or both, sometimes bilaterally, with an area of reference to one or more muscles of the cervical paravertebral musculature; the trapezius is the muscle more frequently involved and, not uncommonly, there is a trigger zone lying outside the painful area [2]. The pain may irradiate to the axilla, to the arm, to the supero-lateral portion of the chest and to the inferior tip of the shoulder blade. It is frequently associated with one of more of the following symptoms: vertigo, tinnitus, diplopia, disphagia. In all such cases the neurological exam is normal.

The pain worsens with movements of the cervical spine or with the strain involved in maintaining a posture.

The mechanism underlying the lesion was extensively studied by different Authors [3]; they all seem to agree that the injury is caused by a flexion-extension vector force, sometimes with a rotational component which follows a sudden and abrupt acceleration-deceleration change, exceeding the biomechanical physiological limits of the cervical spine.

With regard to the mechanism of injury, many different types of traumatic lesions of the cervical spine may be described: hyperflexion and/or hyperextension with or without rotation, sprain or strain, subluxation, dislocation, teardrop fracture, fractures; all of them may singularly occur or be variously associated.

In this work, we will not include those cervical injuries causing a neurological deficit or a definite bony or discal lesion founded on clinical and radiological examinations and involving damage to the spinal cord, the spinal roots or the cervical brachial plexus.

Department of Neuroradiology, IRCSS, Ospedale Maggiore, Via F. Sforza 35, Milano, Italy

The anatomical location of the whiplash injury lies, in our opinion, at muscolo-ligamental level. Consequently, what kind of changes of the cervical spine may be expected to appear at a radiological evaluation in such instances?

The plain standard X-rays projections (antero-posterior, latero-lateral, oblique) obtained with the patient either in standing or sitting position may show a reversal of the physiological lordosis up to a hyperkyphotic appearance, sometimes coexisting with a lateral flexion of the cervical spine due to contraction of the lateral muscles of the neck. In this case, some Authors [3, 4] infer that the spasm of the neck muscle may be very disabling (i.e in children it often reaches the features of a post-traumatic torticollis), especially if unilateral, and may interfere with the postural reflex of the neck ensuing a continuous and annoying vertigo which affects ambulation. Even a sprain to the longissimus colli may be associated with an injury of the cervical sympathetic plexus causing nausea and vertigo [3, 4].

In the lateral projection a widening of the vertebral interspace and perching of the facet joints can be noted due to a lesion of their facetal joint capsule [5]. For this reason, lateral flexion and extension radiographs are useful to demonstrate the possible presence of an abnormal motion of one or more cervical vertebra disclosing injuries of the ligaments complex [6].

When an angular kyphosis is present, then an anterior or posterior subluxation may often be demonstrated and the upper vertebral body is posteriorly or anteriorly displaced. Widening of the distance between the spinous processes (fanning) may be noted due to disruption of the interspinous and posterior ligament [5].

After a congruous period of time, discal and arthrosic modifications develop at the site of the kyphotic angulation.

CT scan has no indication in the evaluation of patient with whiplash syndrome as we defined it here. Although CT allows good visualization of the bony structures, it does not yield a study of the ligamentous complex. CT with 3-D programs may demonstrate bony lesions not otherwise appreciated. It is true, CT permits imaging of the cervical disks and their lesions, however an acute post-traumatic cervical disk herniation is very seldom without neurological deficits [7]. Hence, within the framework of this chapter, CT evaluation is usually normal.

MRI is a relatively recent technique that enables the acquisition, with a single imaging modality, of comprehensive information about the status of the spinal cord. Therefore MRI has became the most important method to evaluate acute severe cervical spinal trauma, now that the initial difficulties, such as patient monitoring during examination, have been overcome.

Nevertheless, the scarcity of MRI units available, the high cost of the exams and the long acquisition time required to obtain a good and thorough imaging make MRI rarely or never used in instances of whiplash syndrome.

However, MRI clearly visualizes the anterior and posterior longitudinal ligaments and the interspinous ligament, hence it is useful in defining their eventual tear. With the appropriate sequences MRI permits evaluation of the soft tissues and the muscles. The presence of edema and/or hemorrhage in such spinal structures produces alteration in the magnetic signal [5, 7, 8].

The principal disadvantage of MRI is the inability to show the cortical bone, making difficult the diagnosis of small fractures or the revelation of displaced bony fragments [5].

In conclusion, we may say that the radiological evaluation of patients complaints related to a whiplash syndrome is somewhat disheartening.

In the acute phase, plain radiographic films may only disclose, in lateral neutral position, a straightening or reversal of the physiological lordosis, or in lateral flexion-extension projection, an increased mobility of the cervical spine. In a selected number of patients, MRI may demonstrate the presence of paravertebral soft tissue edema or hematoma in the muscle of the neck.

At a later date the neutral lateral view may reveal the evolution of a reversed lordosis in an angular kyphosis with the presence of a narrowed intervertebral space and an unco-arthrosis.

However, it can be very difficult to correlate patient's claim with X-ray findings, especially if the radiological evaluation is "normal or almost normal".

Post-traumatic disturbances of the equilibrium (secondary to vertigo, diplopia, tinnitus, headache, etc.) may be present and, in some cases, disabiliting even with a normal radiological examination.

So it may happen that some patients with serious injuries are overlooked or accused of faking, or seeking compensation, while others who are uninjured receive treatment and reward.

References

1. Crowe HE (1928) Injuries to the cervical spine. Presented at the Annual Meeting of the Western Orthopedic Association, San Francisco
2. Cousins MJ, Breidenbough PO eds (1992) Neural blockade. Lippincott, 768-769
3. Bonica JJ (1990) The management of pain. Lea & Febiger 1:854-856
4. Macnab I (1973) The whiplash syndrome. Clin Neurosurg 20:232-241
5. Harris JH, Eideken-Monroe B (1987) The radiology of acute cervical spine trauma. Williams and Wilkins
6. Dosch JC (1985) Trauma. Conventional radiological study in spine injury. Springer Verlag
7. Wimmer B, Hofmann E, Jacob A (1990) Trauma of the spine. CT and MRI. Springer Verlag
8. Grenier N, Halini PH, Frija G, Sigal R (1991) Traumatismes. In: R Sigal, N Grenier, D Doyon, Garcia-Torres E (eds) IRM de la Moelle et du Rachis. Masson

PART 2

PHYSIOPATHOLOGY

Pathophysiology of Whiplash Associated Disorders: Theories and Controversies

M. Magnusson and M. Karlberg

Introduction

The term "whiplash" already suggests difficulties in assessing this problem. Patients suffering from "whiplash" or "whiplash associated disorders" (WAD) are defined as having been exposed to similar types of trauma or sometimes even similar mode of impact, rather than as having a certain type of lesion or set of symptoms [1, 2]. The origin of the term "whiplash" is attributed to H. Crowe [3] who suggested a trauma to the cervico-cranial junction based on the mechanisms of acceleration and deceleration of the head at impact.

Below some different theories of the organic causes of the complaints will be discussed, but it should be pointed out that it would not come as a complete surprise to us if in the future it became apparent that several mechanisms contribute to the complaints of the heterogeneous group of patients suffering from WAD.

Pathophysiologic Mechanisms

There are several different theories to explain the traumatic mechanisms of whiplash injuries, as one has to assume that in such lesions there may be concomitant mild brain injury [4]. The possible pathogeneses may include lesions to the soft tissue of the neck, cervical roots, peripheral and central nervous neuronal tissues, and the inner ear.

Lesions to Soft Tissues of the Neck

On the one hand it has been suggested that WAD should be distinguished from sprained necks, traumatic disk protrusions and damage to cord and nerve roots. On the other hand it is clear that, to associate the symptoms with

Department of Otorhinolaryngology, University Hospital, Lund, Sweden the trauma, the patient should present with neck pain in close connection with the trauma [1, 2]. If the finding that the pain from the neck emanates from the soft tissue and perhaps not from a possible CNS injury as suggested [4], it becomes increasingly difficult to make the suggested separation, especially when considering that the definition of WAD is based on the trauma rather than the lesion [1, 2].

There are generally very few signs of acute structural damage found in X-rays or CT in WAD [1-3]. However, the Quebec Task Force on WAD recommends that X-rays of the cervical columna should be taken in grade II-III WAD, that is, pain associated with musculoskeletal or neurological signs [2]. This would seem to indicate that structural soft tissue or skeletal damage would be uncommon and probably not of importance for the mechanisms behind WAD. However, small even multiple lesions may not be easily recognized on standard X-ray or even CT. Multiple hidden cervical spine lesions have been reported after autopsies of all 22 subjects in a series with skull fractures after traffic accidents and in whom the cervical spines were frozen together with the soft tissues in situ before removal and investigation [5]. Such findings may suggest that, although not found on routine investigations, there may be cervical soft tissue lesions after whiplash injuries. Musculo-skeletal complaints such as tension or tenderness are not uncommon in WAD [1, 2]. Although muscle tension has been suggested to spread from an initial cervical soft tissue lesion [6] and a similar mechanism may be hypothesized to effect proprioception [7], the significance of muscular-skeletal lesions in WAD remains obscure.

Peripheral Nervous Lesions

In whiplash trauma, lesions to the peripheral nervous system have been suggested both to be and not to be of importance [1]. Considering the induced movements of the cervical column during a whiplash trauma it seems possible that there should at least be a risk of traumatic stretching or compression of the peripheral nerves leaving or entering the spine. The importance of such lesions is not known, but it should be pointed out that peripheral nerve lesions have been demonstrated to occasionally produce motor disturbances [8]. Although the mechanisms behind the above observations are not known, it is compelling that peripheral nerve lesions seem to produce such adverse symptoms as parkinsonism [9], tremor [10, 11], and dystonia [10, 12]. Again, the relationship between peripheral nerve lesions and WAD is not known.

Central Nervous System Lesions

Neuro-imaging techniques have failed to report visible structural damage after whiplash injuries [13]. This has been taken as evidence that whiplash trauma does not produce significant cerebral lesions [1]. The same may be said for mild brain injuries [4]. The cervical trauma resulting from a whiplash injury often coincides with a significant acceleration-deceleration of or even direct impact to the head, which can be suspected to produce mild traumatic brain injuries. Furthermore, some of the symptoms of WAD are similar or identical to those of mild traumatic brain injuries and post-concussional syndromes. For example attention deficits, concentration disturbances, fatigue and sleep disturbances as well as depression, anxiety and pain are common findings [4, 14]. Diffuse axonal injury produced by shear forces generated during acceleration-deceleration of the nervous tissue is considered to constitute the primary pathophysiologic cause of traumatic brain injuries [15] especially to the parasagittal white matter [16].

Decreased attention is a major result of mild traumatic brain injuries and is also considered to cause concomitant cognitive deficits [4]. The decreased attentiveness may remain for a longer period depending upon the age of the patient [17] and may not be completely restored even after years. Especially demanding work situations, fatigue or other disorders may unveil the imperfect recovery.

An alternative pathophysiologic mechanism causing central nervous lesions in whiplash injuries has been suggested by Portnoy in the monkey and Svensson in the pig [18, 19]. During the intense deceleration of the head there is a fast and short rise of the intracranial and also intraspinal cerebrospinal fluid pressure, approaching values as high as 150 mm Hg. The authors argue that such a pressure peak may cause damage to the neural tissue and be responsible for the concomitant symptoms. Again the validity of the hypothesis remains to be tested further.

Vestibular Lesions

Several investigators report a high frequency of abnormal central vestibular signs in patients with whiplash injuries [14]. Peripheral vestibular injuries, especially perilymphatic fistulas, have recently been suggested as possible causes of some symptoms in WAD [20]. WAD patients do not generally present with sudden deafness or pronounced hearing losses immediately after a trauma. Such findings would have been expected if oval or round window ruptures would be common in WAD.

50

Discussion

There is no consensus about the pathophysiological mechanisms of whiplash or WAD. Taking the above reasoning into consideration it seems not impossible that combinations of CNS lesions and soft tissue or peripheral neural lesions might enhance each other or coincide to produce the diverse set of symptoms that one might encounter in these patients. Furthermore, a disturbed attention span may result in different sets of cognitive impairments, concentration deficits and fatigue. Long-standing pain may also trigger psychiatric conditions. WAD per se seems to evoke psychiatric conditions such as anxiety and depression [14]. Although it is unclear to what extent this is due to the lesion itself or secondary to other symptoms, these psychiatric impairments may by themselves contribute to the distress of the patient.

Although entirely hypothetical, it is intriguing to consider the abundance of attention and concentration deficits, loss of stamina, and personality changes reported by these patients and to compare these patients to those with mild lesions to the ventro-medial prefrontal cortex or cingulate area [21], especially considering the preference for parasagittal white matter lesions in traumatic brain injuries.

The possibilities of malingering or enhancing ones' symptoms to receive medico-legal benefits have not been discussed here. It should only be pointed out that it is the authors' opinion that such a possibility should be neither forgotten nor overemphasized. At present we have to conclude that we do not have a specific unifying pathophysiological explanation of WAD. Further research as well as an open but careful attitude in considering the problem are both needed.

References

1. Pearce JMS (1994) Polemics of chronic whiplash injury. Neurology 44:1993-1997
2. Spitzer WO, Skovron ML, Salmi LR, Cassidy JD, Duranceau J, Suissa S, Zeiss E (1995) Scientific monograph of the Quebec Task Force on whiplash-associated disorders. Spine [Suppl]:20
3. Crowe H (1928) Injuries to the cervical spine. Presentation to the annual meeting of the Western Orthopedic Association, San Francisco
4. Alexander MP (1995) Mild traumatic brain injury: pathophysiology, natural history, and clinical management. Neurology 45:1253-1260
5. Jónsson H, Bring G, Rauschning W, Sahlstedt B (1991) Hidden cervical spine injuries in traffic accident victims with skull fractures. J Spinal Disorders 4:251-263
6. Johansson H, Sojka P (1991) Pathophysiological mechanisms involved in genesis and spread of muscular tension in occupational muscle pain and in chronic musculoskeletal pain syndromes: a hypothesis. Med Hypoth 35:196-203

7. Karlberg M (1995) The neck and human balance. Thesis. Lund, Sweden

8. Jankovic J (1994) Post traumatic movement disorders: central and peripheral mechanisms. Neurology 44:2006-2014

9. Schott GD (1986) Induction of involuntary movements by peripheral trauma. An analogy with causalgia. Lancet 2:712-716

10. Jankovic J, Van der Linden C (1988) Dystonia and tremor induced by peripheral trauma: predisposing factors. J Neurol Neurosurg Psychiatry 51:l512-1519

11. Cole JD, Illis LS, Sedgewick EM (1989) Unilateral essential tremor after wrist immobilization: a case report. J Neurol Neurosurg Psychiatry 52:286-287

12. Bhatia KK, Bhatt MH, Marsden CD (1993) The causalgia-dystonia syndrome. Brain 116:843-851

13. Yarnell PR, Rossie GV (1988) Minor whiplash head injury with major debilitation. Brain Inj 273:255-258

14. Ettlin TM, Kischka U, Reichmann S, Radii EW, Heim S, Wengen D, Benson F (1993) Cerebral symptoms after whiplash injury of the neck: a prospective clinical and neuropsychological study of whiplash injury. J Neurol Neurosurg Psychiatry 55:943-948

15. Povlishock JT, Becker DP, Cheng CLY et al (1986) Axonal change in minor head injury. J Neuropathol Exp Neurol 42:225-242

16. Gennarelli TA, Thibault LE, Adams JH et al (1982) Diffuse axonal injury and traumatic coma in the primate. Ann Neurol 12:564-574

17. Binder LM (1986) Persisting symptoms after mild head injury: a review of the postconcussive syndrome. J Clin Exp Neuropsychol 8:32

18. Portnoy HD, Benjamin D, Brian, M, McCoy LE, Prince B, Edgerton R, Young J (1970) Intracranial pressure and head acceleration during whiplash. Proc 14th STAPP Car Crash Conf, SAE paper n. 700900, SAE Inc, USA, LC 67-22372 3-346

19. Svennson MY (1993) Neck Injuries in rear-end car collisions. Thesis, Chalmers University of Technology, Gothenburg, Sweden

20. Chester JB Jr (1991) Whiplash, postural control, and the inner ear. Spine 16(7):716-720

21. Damasio A (1994) Descartes error. Picador

Postural Studies on Whiplash Injuries

P. M. GAGEY

The postural study of whiplash victims, seen at the Institut de Posturologie, raises several questions that merit discussion. Why does the great majority of patients present with a disharmonious postural syndrome? What is the significance of a fundamental oscillation of their stabilometric signals at 0.2 Hz? Is there any particular significance to the asymmetrical electromyographic activity of neck muscles in these patients? What place must be made for the anatomical lesion of the cervical spine among the diagnostic criteria of post-traumatic cervical syndrome?

We will focus our attention on each of these questions, one-by-one.

Disharmonious Postural Syndrome

The search for an abnormal postural tonic asymmetry forms the basis of the clinical postural examination. We look for this asymmetry at the level of the axial musculature by means of movements that obey the laws of spinal movement, Lowett's laws (1907) - cited and disseminated by Fryette [1] - for example, during the lateral inclination of the spine of the subject standing up. According to Lowett's laws, this movement is accompanied by a contralateral rotation of the lumbar and dorsal vertebrae, easily perceived by gently placing one's hands on the patient's iliac wings and scapulae, while he leans sidewards.

We explore distal musculature by means of Fukuda's stepping test [2], with measurement of neck-reflex gains [3].

When the muscle tone is abnormally asymmetrical, we can speak of a "postural syndrome": it is said to be "harmonious" when the hypertonicity is crossed between the axial and distal musculatures; in the opposite case, the postural syndrome is said to be "disharmonious". Barré's "vertical" provides a visual summary of these postural syndrome analyses (Fig. 1).

The overwhelming majority of whiplash victims present a disharmonious postural syndrome; this surprisingly high incidence of disharmonious pos-

Institut de Posturologie, Av. de Corbera 4, Paris, France

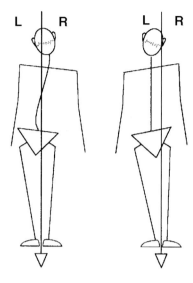

Fig. 1. Harmonious and disharmonious postural syndromes. *On the left,* in harmonious syndrome, the hypertonicity of the axial and distal muscles is crossed. *On the right,* in disharmonious postural syndrome, the hypertonicity of the axial and distal muscles is homolateral. (From [3])

tural syndrome following whiplash is statistically significant.

What does it mean? Uemura and Cohen [4] showed that by localized destruction of the vestibular nuclei in the monkey it was possible to induce harmonious or disharmonious postural syndromes depending upon the level of the lesion. However, it is difficult to imagine that whiplash systematically produces a lesion of the vestibular nuclei and even more difficult to think that such a lesion would always occur at the same site. Thus, the meaning of a disharmonious postural syndrome must be sought elsewhere.

A clear-cut asymmetry of the electric activity of the neck muscles almost always exists following whiplash and this does not seem strange when we remember the incidence of cervical articulation lesions caused by this type of trauma. The muscles contract to mitigate the consequences of rupturing ligaments. Could this tonic - organic asymmetry of the neck muscles be the origin of the disharmonious postural syndrome of whiplash victims? The hypothesis, as yet unproven, is interesting because it emphasizes the postural importance of these muscles, "the veritable braces of the head and neck that act as spatial positioners of the otolithic and visual reference points", according to Boquet's terminology [3].

In addition, the postural importance of these neck muscles is directly demonstrated by stabilometric recordings of these patients: clear-cut, statistically significant asymmetry of the areas of the statokinesigrams appears between the recordings made with the head turned to the right and then to the left (Fig. 2).

The Fundamental Oscillation at 0.2 Hz

Frequency analysis of the stabilometric signals of whiplash victims using the Fourier transform leads very often to the appearance of a fundamental oscillation around 0.2 Hz (Fig. 3). This fundamental oscillation at 0.2 Hz appears equally on recordings made with the eyes open or closed.

This 0.2 Hz fundamental oscillation must not be confused with the fundamental oscillation at 0.3 Hz described by Taguchi [5]. The 0.3 Hz frequency corresponds to the resonance frequency of the inverted human pendulum that appears during dysregulations of the fine postural control system of which it is sometimes the only stabilometric witness. This fundamental oscillation simply demonstrates that the postural system is no longer able to damp out this resonance frequency of the human pendulum and lets it pass.

The 0.2 Hz fundamental oscillation has a completely different significance. We showed that a population of patients suffering from rachialgia is characterized by a peak at the frequency of 0.2 Hz, when the mean power spectrum is compared to that of a population of normal subiects [6]. However, this fundamental oscillation is not pathognomonic of a rachidian disorder; it has another origin.

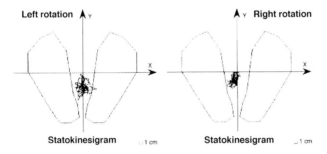

Left rotation ↑ y   ↑ y Right rotation

Statokinesigram   ⌐ 1 cm   Statokinesigram   ⌐ 1 cm

Fig. 2. Stabilometric recordings with the head turned to the left and the right. *On the left*, the subject's head was turned to the left during the recording session: the area of the statokinesigram is 2.092 mm^2. *On the right*, the subject's head was rotated to the right during the recording session: the area of the statokinesigram is 867 mm^2. The ration of the areas or the cervical quotient is statistically significant: 2.41 ($p < 0.05$)

Fig. 3. Fourier's transform of the stabilometric signals of a whiplash victim. The fundamental oscillation is evident, clearly separated, at a frequency band of about 0.2 Hz. (From [3])

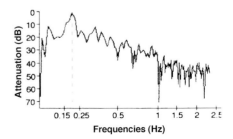

The respiration rhythm is situated in this frequency band of 0.2 Hz; it does not appear [7] or appears only slightly [8] on the stabilograms of normal standing subjects. Gurfinkel and Elner [7] suggest the possibility of a postural adjustment in preparation of the act of breathing that corrects in advance the postural perturbations resulting from movements of the thoracic cage.

It seems important to emphasize the incidence of the appearance of this respiratory rhythm on the stabilograms of subjects with a rachidian dysfunction, because Tardy [9] showed very close relationships between the static spinal musculature and the muscles involved in respiration.

Asymmetry of the Electromyographic Activity of the Neck Muscles

For many years, Boquet and Boismare [10] studied comparatively the electromyograph (EMG) of the superior heads of the trapezius muscles, left and right. In whiplash victims they almost always found marked asymmetry of these EMGs, with the patient's head in either the normal position (Fig. 4) or between positions with the head turned to the left and to the right (Fig. 5).

What is most remarkable on the EMG tracings of these patients is not only the asymmetry but also the amplitude of electrical activity. Boquet

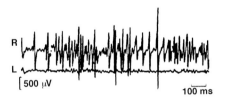

Fig. 4. Electromyograph (EMG) of neck muscles. EMG of the superior heads of the right and left trapezius muscles of a whiplash victim with his head in the normal position. The asymmetry of the tracings is obvious. (From [3])

Fig. 5. Electromyograph (EMG) of neck muscles. EMG of the superior heads of the right (*uneven numbers*) and left (*even numbers*) trapezius muscles. *1-2*: head in the normal position; *3-4*: head turned to the right; *5-6*: head turned to the left. The asymmetry appears when the head is rotated towards the right. (From [3])

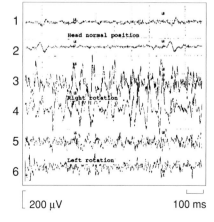

noted signs of increased levels of vigilance, emotionalism and basic anxiety in these patients. All whiplash victims do not necessarily have postural disorders. A supplementary factor is required which Boquet and Boismare link to this hypervigilance, that is, anxious individuals very often have neck pains and they blame it on early arthritis, but wrongly so, because one sees people with arthritis sufficiently severe to generate cracking sounds who do not suffer and do not have contractures, but are calm individuals. This clinical contrast underlines the increased reactivity of neck neuromuscular spindles when the vigilance level is heightened [10]. This brings to mind the fundamental studies that demonstrated the noradrenergic innervation of the neuromuscular spindles [11, 12] and, more generally, the influence of the autonomous nervous system on the postural system [13].

Lesions of the Cervical Spine

Treatment of post-traumatic cervical syndrome by strictly postural techniques (optical prisms, stimulation soles) has been a failure. But clinical posturology has taught us that, with every failure of postural treatments, a poorly understood lesion must be sought. This is indeed the case, well-established today, for mandibular lesions responsible for craniomandibular dysfunctions; we now know that the latter must be treated prior to initiating any postural therapy. This is also true for irritative lesions of plantar pressure points that are able to generate distant postural dysfunction; these lesions must be dealt with first. This hierarchy of treatments is easily explained: prisms and stimulation soles can only modify sensory integration. Addressing the lesion takes precedence over the subtleties of improving sensory integration.

Nowadays, lesions of the cervical spine after whiplash are far from always being poorly understood; medical imaging techniques have made enormous progress. Even before the era of computed tomography scanners and magnetic resonance imaging, Gentaz et al. [14], by multiplying the dynamic projections for radiography of the cervical spine, had detected obvious signs of cervical sprain, e.g. rupture of the continuity of the posterior wall of the vertebral bodies (Fig. 6) or overlapping of posterior articulations.

Normally, the posterior faces of the vertebral bodies remain perfectly aligned, even during hyperflexion and hyperextension of the neck. When a step-like shift appears in this posterior wall (between C3 and C4 in the drawing on the right of Fig. 6), a ligament has been torn, the neck sprained. These shifts usually only appear in dynamic positions, in this case, hyperextension.

Discovery of a cervical lesion subsequent to whiplash seems so important that we are tempted to say that no diagnosis of post-traumatic cervical syndrome can be made in its absence, especially when the whiplash is not recent. As long as the lesion is not found, it must be sought with perseverance.

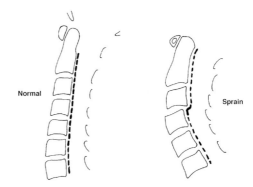

Fig. 6. Posterior walls, normal
and after cervical sprain

If, despite the multiplication of tests, the lesion is not seen, the diagnosis
should remain highly suspect. The neck is the privileged site of expression
of all sorts of "distant" pathologies, for example, oculomotor - strabismal
torticollis, occlusive, spinal and even plantar - that have nothing to do with
whiplash. The cervical spine is a trap for the clinician.

Treatment

It is useless to apply postural techniques to treat a whiplash victim with a
cervical sprain. Therapy of the lesion takes precedence over attempts to
manipulate sensory integration.

In contrast, Boquet and Boismare [10] insist upon the necessity to treat
from the start the excessive anxiety, translated as permanent neurectasia, of
these patients. The recommended therapeutic strategy is myoresolutive and
sedative. The treatment starts with a diazepam (20 mg/ml) drip, in combination with α- and β-blockers that reduce the activity of the autonomous nervous system. The dosages are adjusted until the desired levels of vigilance
and muscular tonus are obtained for each subject. Once the patient is "relaxed", work can begin on the neck.

Conclusion

For more than 100 years, since the studies of Longet, we have known that
the neck muscles are involved in postural control and we confirm this knowledge every day in whiplash victims. However, over the past few years, our
attention has been drawn towards the overall level of vigilance of these patients that must be taken into account before starting therapy.

We are also better able to explore the traps posed by the cervical spine,
where numerous postural tonic pathologies can express themselves without

any local lesion. These observations lead us to insist upon searching signs of cervical sprain using all available means of medical imaging before settling on a diagnosis of whiplash.

The discovery of a cervical lesion is extremely important for determining the therapeutic strategy - it formally counterindicates the use of any postural techniques.

References

1. Fryette HH (1978) Principes des techniques ostéopathiques. Maloine, Paris
2. Fukuda T (1959) The stepping test. Two phases of the labyrinthine reflex. Acta Otolaryngol, Stockh, 50:95-108
3. Gagey PM, Weber B (1995) Posturologie; régulations et dérèglements de la station debout. Masson, Paris
4. Uemura T, Cohen B (1973) Effects of vestibular nuclei lesions on vestibulo-ocular reflexes and posture in monkeys. Acta Otolaryngol, Stockh [Suppl. 315]
5. Taguchi K (1978) Spectral analysis of the movement of the center of gravity in vertiginous and ataxic patients. Agressologie 19B:69-70
6. Gagey PM (1986) Postural disorders among workers on building sites. In: Bles W, Brandt Th (eds). Disorders of posture and gait. Elsevier, Amsterdam, 253-268
7. Gurfinkel VS, Elner AM (1968) The relation of stability in a vertical posture to respiration in focal cerebral lesions of different etiology. Neuropathol Psychiatry, 58:1014-1018 (in russian)
8. Bouisset S, Duchêne JL (1994) Is body balance more perturbed by respiration in seating than in standing posture? Neuro Report 5:957-960
9. Tardy D (1992) Systèmes moteurs posturaux du tronc, vieillissement, déclin. Critique de la Posturologie, Association Française de Posturologie, Paris, 52:1-9
10. Boquet J, Boismare F (1982) Étude physiopathologique du syndrome cervical post-traumatique. Rôle du tonus végétatif. Rev F Dommage Corpor 8:397-410
11. Hunt CC, Jame L, Laporte Y (1982) Effects of stimulating the lumbar sympathetic trunk on cat hindlimb muscle spindles. Arch Ital Biol 120:371-384
12. Grassi C, Perin F, Artusio E, Passatore M (1993) Modulation of the jaw jerk reflex by the sympathetic nervous system. Arch Ital Biol 131:213-226
13. Camis M (1928) Fisiologia dell'appparato vestibolare. Zanichelli, Bologna
14. Gentaz R, Gagey PM, Goumot J, Rouquet Y, Baron JB (1975) La radiographie du rachis cervical au cours du syndrome post-commotionnel. Agressologie 16A:33-46

Whiplash Effects on Hypothalamus and the Sympathetic System

R. BONIVER

Introduction

The so-called posterior cervical sympathetic syndrome of Barré is a disputed cause of vertigo arising from cervical lesions. Barré (1924) proposed that cervical lesions might irritate the sympathetic vertebral plexus and result in a decreased blood flow to the labyrinth due to constriction of the internal auditory artery. Although numerous clinical reports of Barré syndrome have been published, few objective data exist to support an association between episodic vertigo and cervical sympathetic dysfunction. Since intracranial circulation is autoregulated independently of cervical sympathetic control, it is unlikely that lesions in the vertebrosympathetic plexus could produce focal constriction of the vasculature to the inner ear.

Hinoki, first in 1971 and in detail in 1985, proposed an hypothesis in which hypothalamus took a fundamental place to explain vertigo due to whiplash injury.

The Hypothalamus

The hypothalamus is unquestionably of great significance both phylogenetically and anthropologically. It plays striking roles in many aspects of mammalian physiology. It undoubtedly contains integrative mechanisms which, in addition to their effect on behaviour patterns, also aid in regulating the basic life functions of the organism. However, this integration is apparently carried out through its relationship with other parts of the nervous system, including the so-called higher levels, as well as through the endocrine system.

It is in this field of interrelationship that some of the most pressing problems lie. It must be appreciated that while this interesting region of the brain is only part of a system of complex circuits, it is an extremely important link

Maître de Conférences, Université de Liège, Rue de Bruxelles 21 - B-4800 Verviers, Tel. 87-221760, Fax 87-224608 in these circuits and is so strategically placed that its derangement may have profound effects.

It is important that the hypothalamus be regarded as part of a series of complex neural circuits involving brain stem, cerebral hemisphere and other parts of the diencephalon. These circuits are poorly understood, but evidence for rich connections with septal, subcallosal, preoptic and frontotemporal areas has been offered.

The hypothalamus is considered to be the most rostral portion of the reticular formation and similarly is poorly differentiated with the exception of the magnocellular neurosecretory system. The hypothalamus is also the most caudal aspect of the limbic system and thus the brain region through which limbic system output comes to control autonomic and endocrine function. The paraventricular nucleus of the hypothalamus (PVN) is one of the most vascularised areas of the brain. The PVN distinguishes itself from other hypothalamic nuclei in that it plays the dominant role in neuronally coupling autonomic, endocrine, and somatomotor responses to environmental stressors.

It accomplishes this through a rich network of innervation from the forebrain, limbic system, other hypothalamic nuclei, and brain stem autonomic centres such as the nucleus of the solitary tract and the dorsal vagal complex. PVN innervates median eminence, pituitary, brain stem nuclei, and spinal cord.

Concentrations in epinephrine (EPI) in the para-ventricular nucleus in human hypothalamus are rather high (Mefford et al. 1978). If stressful motion was shown to lead to a significant rise in EPI and norepinephrine (NE), then this rise would be different from subject to subject and would therefore be more prominent in subjects more resistant to motion sickness. Strangely enough, in those cases, no correlations were found between measured levels of ACTH and EPI even though EPI exerts a stimulatory influence on the pituary gland's release of ACTH. It is well known that ACTH and smaller peptides like ACTH 4-10 reduce latency in recovery of normal sensorimotor functions following unilateral labyrinthectomy.

Corticotropin release factor (CRF) - containing neurons have been found in the medial vestibular nucleus and may contribute to CRF - containing climbing fibers shown to project from the inferior olive to the cerebellum.

Hinoki's Hypothesis

According to Hinoki, patients with whiplash injury present with an hypertonicity of the soft supporting tissues of the neck due to the overexcitation of the cervical proprioceptors, which is caused by an excitation of sympathical beta-receptors in the muscle spindles. He has demonstrated the development of granular vescles at the end of unmyelinated nerve fibers near motor nerve endings of these spindles.

Abnormal centripetal impulses arising from the injured cervical soft tissues may ascend along the spinoreticular tract to the brain stem. Among the ascending pathways from the cervical and lumbar proprioceptors to the brain stem, the spinoreticular tract seems to be the most important, since most of its fibers ascend along the lateral fasciculus and the anterior column and terminate in the reticular formation of both the medulla oblongata and the pons. However, some fibers of this tract ascend directly to the midbrain and are connected to Deiter's nucleus.

Furthermore, this tract changes neurons in the medulla oblongata, the pons and the midbrain and terminates in the superior colliculus. It is generally accepted that the reticular formation of these parts of the brain, as well as Deiter's nucleus and the superior colliculus, are active in both ocular and spinal reflexes related to body equilibrium. Among the descending paths from the brain stem, the median longitudinal fasciculus (MLF) is important in cases of vertigo, because this tract originates in the brain stem and is connected to both the oculomotor nuclei and the somatomotor cells in the ventral column. The reticulospinal tract also originates in the brain stem reticular formation of both the medulla oblongata and the pons and is connected to the somatomotor cells in the ventral column. This tract is thought to have a close relationship with the spinoreticular tract mentioned above. Thus, the MLF and the reticulospinal tract seem especially important in the development of disequilibrium because of whiplash injury. The hypothalamus must also play an important role in producing vertigo due to whiplash injury, since most of Hinoki patients, with vertigo following whiplash injury, had various autonomic symptoms, such as lacrimation, abnormal sweating and palpitation.

The cerebellum is, of course, involved in the development of this type of vertigo, since it is closely connected to the proprioceptors of the cervical and lumbar regions as well as to the brain stem (Fig. 1).

After several experiments, Hinoki further demonstrated that the abnormal autonomic reactions in patients with whiplash injury were not due to the irritation of the injured posterior cervical sympathetic nerves but to overstimulation of the proprioceptor of the neck.

On the basis of their report and the known fiber connections in the central nervous system, it may be assumed that in patients with whiplash injury, delayed pupil constriction in response to light is probably because of overstimulation of a sympathetic component in the hypothalamo-brain stem system brought about by centripetal impulses from the injured proprioceptors of the neck and waist. In addition, the spinoreticular tract is probably involved in the conduction of these impulses, since this tract ascends along the lateral fasciculus and the anterior column in the cervical and lumbar cords

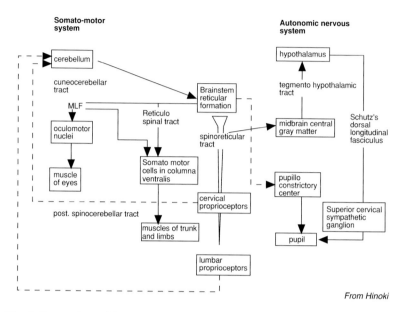

Fig. 1. Connections of lumbar and cervical proprioceptors within the somato-motor system

and terminates in both the reticular formation of the brain stem and the central gray matter of the midbrain.

The central gray matter of the midbrain is then connected to the hypothalamus both through the tegmento-hypothalamic tract and diffuse ascending neurons. There is evidence to support this assumption, since Hinoki found that, in patients with delayed pupil constriction in response to light, ataxia of the eyes and body tended to be aggravated by the subcutaneous injection of adrenaline.

Moreover, Kawamura and Oshuma (1962) reported that adrenaline acts directly on the posterior hypothalamus, an important center of the sympathetic nervous system. Okada et al. (1960) also reported that in cats the electrical activities of the short ciliary nerves, which are involved in pupil constriction, were significantly decreased by the injection of adrenaline. According to their explanation, over-stimulation of the hypothalamus induced by adrenaline suppresses the activity of the pupillo-constrictory center of the midbrain, leading to pupil dilatation.

To summarize, the over excitation of the arrival proprioceptors should be because of an hypersensitivity to sympathetical stimulation, inducing central disturbances by afferent nervous pathways at the level of brain stem, cerebellar and hypothalamus, affecting the oculomotor system and gait control.

Conclusion

To sustain Hinoki's hypothesis it was demonstrated:
- The existence in the hypothalamus of neurons with high sensitivity to catecholamines and the correlation between alteration of EEG and stimulation of neck proprioceptors.
- The presence of beta-receptors into the brain stem, including pontine reticular structures. (Stampacchia et al. 1988).
- The influence of injection of drugs stimulating beta-receptors in muscles of the neck on the disturbances of EMG and OPK recordings.
- The influence of cervical roots sections or injection of procaine of muscle on the gait.

But, following whiplash injury, in humans, NE or EPI levels in the blood have a great variability and are not in correlation with cortical secretion because of this stress. The symptoms are very variable.

To have a perfect demonstration of Hinoki's hypothesis, it would be interesting to correlate the modification of the EMG and OPK testings with the modification of cortical activation, NE and EPI levels in the blood and the symptoms of the patients.

References

1. Barré JA (1926) Sur un syndrome sympathique cervical postérieur et sa cause fréquente: l'arthrite cervicale. Revue Neurol 33:1246-1294
2. Hinoki M (1985) Vertigo due to whiplash injury: a neuro-otological approach. Acta Otolaryngol, Stockholm [Suppl 419]:9-29
3. Hinoki M, Hine S, Tada Y (1971) Neurootological study on vertigo due to whiplash injury. Equil Res [Suppl 1]:5-29
4. Kawamura H, Oshima K (1962) Effect of adrenaline on the hypothalamic activating system. Jap J Physiol 12:225-233
5. Mefford IN, Oke A, Keller R, Adams RM, Jonsson G (1978) Epinephrine distribution in human brain. Neurosc Lett 9:277-287
6. Okada H, Nakano O, Nishida I (1960) Effects of sciatic stimulation upon the efferent impulses in the long ciliary nerves of the cat. Jap J Physiology 10:327-337
7. Stampacchia G, D'ascanio P, Hoin E, Pompeiano O (1988) Gain regulation of the vestibulospinal reflex following microinjection of a beta-adrenergic agonist or antagonist in to the locus coeruleus and the dorsal pontine reticular formation. Adv Oto Rhino Laryng 41:134-141

Whiplash Effects on the Vestibulo-oculomotor System

L. M. Ödkvist

Introduction

For balancing, motor control and keeping visual objects steady on the retina, the vestibular system and the interaction with the visual system is of paramount importance. Balance is maintained via cooperation between the vestibular afferents, proprioception, podalic pressure receptors and vision [1]. For diagnostics postural tests are important but the easiest and most accurate way to study the vestibular system is recording of spontaneous and provoked eye movements, and the interaction with the visual system. Often the cause for vertigo can be unveiled with these methods. For eye movement recording video or photoelectric devices may be used but the most widely used method is electronystagmography (ENG) [14].

The Vestibulo-oculomotor Reflex

Examination of ocular movements in response to stimulation of the vestibular part of the inner ear is important for evaluation of the state of the vestibular system in patients. The vestibulo-ocular reflex (VOR) connects the sensory transducers, the hair cells in the semicircular canals and the otolithic organs in the vestibular part of the labyrinth with the extrinsic ocular muscles. Stimulation of the inner ears results in movements of the eyes. With VOR, during head movements the visual target is always centered on the fovea. Vestibular stimulation is achieved either by rotatory movements of the head, or in the caloric test, thermal irrigation of the ear canal. The advantage of the caloric test is that it tests each labyrinth separately. Caloric irrigation is, however, a crude and unphysiological stimulus. The rotatory test, on the other hand, uses a more physiological stimulus, however exciting both ears simultaneously.

Department of Otolaryngology, University Hospital, S-58185 Linköping, Sweden, Tel. (46)-13-222000, Fax (46)-13-222504

Vestibulo-visual Interaction

The directioning of the eyes is a function of the cooperation of the vestibular organs, neck proprioception and vision. In cases of conflict the visual reflexes override VOR at least in the low frequency area. In high frequency swings the ocular motion is driven mainly by VOR. The cerebellar flocculus and nodulus mediate the interaction. Patients with cerebellar lesions may have a defunct visual suppression ability. Some patients with brainstem lesions may have the same functional defect. The neck proprioceptors also help maintain gaze direction during movements of the neck, body and towards visible targets. There is a strong confluence of cervical, visual, and vestibular afferents in the vestibular brainstem nuclei. For examining the patient with vertigo or balance disorder, eye movement investigation is mandatory, perferably using ENG.

VOR Examination - The Caloric Test

A thermic stimulation of the labyrinth is usually achieved using water with a temperature 7° above or below body temperature. The patient lies down with the head elevated 30° from horizontal. The test is based on the fact that the caloric stimulation induces a movement of the endolymph in the semicircular canals [3]. A nystagmus is elicited and calculated concerning different qualities of the reaction. Sometimes the duration of the nystagmus response is recorded but the most valid parameter is the speed of the slow phase of the elicited nystagmus beats. The duration of the reaction is an uncertain measurement of the caloric response and can be normal although a diminished caloric response may be present, which is unveiled only by measuring the speed of the slow phase of the nystagmus beat. The equipment needed is not expensive nor complicated. However the caloric response has severe limitations. Because of individual differences in the temporal bone anatomy as well as differences in the local temporal bone blood flow, the temperature gradients can be quite variable. The recording and calculation of the caloric response need ENG [2]. The frequency of beats per unit time is closely related to labyrinthine activity and is another parameter that could be used. However practical experience and the international literature suggest that the parameter to be used is the speed of the slow component, usually 10°-25°/s at the maximum of the response. Hot and cold water should be used, i.e. a total of four irrigations are needed, which allows calculation of not only the side difference but also the directional preponderance defined as the sum of nystagmus reaction in one direction compared to the sum in the other direction. A difference in directional preponderance of up to 30% is the normal limit. A side difference between the right and the left ear of 20% is the upper normal limit.

Rotatory Tests

Rotatory testing has been in use since the turn of the century. The main drawback with the rotatory test is that the stimulation affects both labyrinths simultaneously. The equipment for rotatory testing is usually expensive and complicated. One advantage with the rotatory test is that the eye movement responses are not dependent on the individual anatomical variations and the recordings can be performed on subjects who do not tolerate caloric irrigation. One additional advantage is that rotatory test provides a natural physiological acceleration stimulus. Different stimulus patterns have been used in rotatory testing - trapezoidal, triangular and damped sinusoidal. Sinusoidal stimulation produces alternating endolymph movements in the two inner ears, imitating normal head movements. A sinusoidal stimulus is characterised by frequency and amplitude of the accelerations. The new method in the field of vestibular testing is sinusoidal rotatory chairs driven by highly controllable motors combined with modern recording techniques.

A vast amount of data has been collected from rotatory testing using broad frequency swings (0.5-5 Hz) [4, 10, 18]. The slow sinusoidal harmonic acceleration test uses swings in the frequency range of 0.01-0.16 Hz with a peak velocity of 50°/s and an acceleration from 3° to 50°/s^2. In low frequency harmonic acceleration testing there are difficulties in testing compensatory eye movements. The effect of alertness level was found to be extremely important. A very low gain could leave a false impression of bilateral vestibular deficiency making interpretations difficult. It could be concluded from a study [12] that eye movements elicited by rotation are not solely the result of the VOR, but caused by the influence of vestibular input, central processing, habituation, and mental sets based on visual input.

The autorotation test, an interesting VOR test, uses the equipment for ENG but the patient himself sinusoidally turns the head to the right and left rhythmically [17]. A calculation is made of the difference between the head movements and the eye movements. The equipment is inexpensive and easy to handle but the drawback is that cervical influences cannot be avoided. Thus the test is not useful in cases of cervical vertigo or whiplash injuries.

The Head Shaking Test

A simple way of testing the vestibulo-oculomotor system is to have the patient shake his head with a frequency of 1-2 Hz for 10 s. Immediately after stopping the movement, eye movements are observer under Frenzel glasses or preferably recorded by ENG. A post head shake nystagmus for several seconds indicates that there is an asymmetry in the peripheral or central part of the vestibular sytem [11].

Neck Torsion Nystagmus

In some cases of neck lesions a simple turning of the head to the right or left may elicit a nystagmus, which can be studied preferably with ENG. Cervical influence on the vestibulo-oculomotor system may also be unveiled if the patient is sitting in a swing chair, the head is held steady by the examiner and the eye movements are observed while the chair with the patient is turned rythmically clockwise and counterclockwise.

Otolith Testing

The otolithic organs in the sacculus and utriculus are transducers of linear acceleration, e.g. gravity. Eccentric rotatory testing can unveil unilateral or bilateral function loss in the otolithic organs. During the rotation the subject experiences an illusion of tilt and in the darkness places a bias light bar at an angle to true horizontal and even has a tilt of the eyeballs. This type of investigation is rather new and still not fully validated [5, 8].

Visual Suppression

The vestibulo-ocular reflex cancelling or visual suppression mechanism can be tested during the caloric response in darkness when a lamp is lit for 10 s, allowing ocular fixation. The induced eye movement speed should decrease to 30% of its value in darkness (Fig 1). The visual suppression test becomes even more sensitive if it is performed in the rotatory chair with the instruction to the patient to fixate on a target by moving with the chair [6, 7, 9, 16] (Fig 2).

The patient is asked to fixate on a dot on a frame mounted on the chair which is placed directly in front of the eyes. ENG is performed and the eye movements are compared by computer with the head movements. The visual suppression test when performed in this way is a sensitive tool in the diagnosis of cerebellar and brainstem function disturbances.

Ocular Smooth Pursuit

The human eye can follow an object moving over the field of vision up to an angular speed of approximately 60°/s. This can be tested with ENG. The mechanism uses the visual system and oculomotor relay stations in the cerebellum, cerebrum and brainstem. CNS lesions may be unveiled using the smooth pursuit test, looking for low gains or jerks in the eye movements.

68

Cal. 30°C right Visual suppression

S.L.

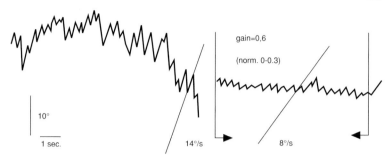

gain=0,6

(norm. 0-0.3)

10°

1 sec.

14°/s

8°/s

Fig. 1. Pathological visual suppression in a patient with a brain stem lesion. In darkness the speed of the slow component is 14°/s and with visual fixation 8°/s indicating pathologically high gain

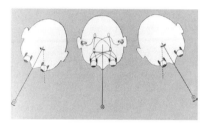

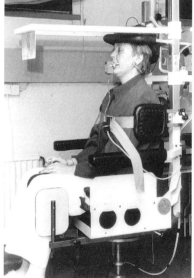

Fig. 2. Visual suppression test in the rotatory chair. Head movements are recorded with the accelerometer on the biteboard. Eye movements are recorded with electronystagmography. The instruction is to fixate on the dot on the screen moving by the chair. Thus the target is always right in front of the eyes

Visual suppression and the smooth pursuit are used for the same purpose, namely to keep the visual target on the fovea. The condition for the two systems is, however, somewhat different as the pursuit system mainly functions when the visual surrounding is in motion and the visual suppression system is operative when the VOR is stimulated by head movements. In a series of investigations [16], certain patients presented with pathology in both tests whereas with others, positive results were seen in the smooth pursuit test alone, indicating that the two systems are not identical, which had been suggested earlier. Figure 3 shows the results from a patient with a cerebellar angioma with pathology in the pursuit system as well as in the visual suppression system. Even in healthy volunteers indications could be found that the two systems are not identical. In particular a comparison between sinusoidal and pseudorandomized movement patterns revealed that prediction was more marked in the pursuit than in the suppression mechanism (Fig. 4). Both tests are capable of detecting pathology in the posterior fossa [13, 15].

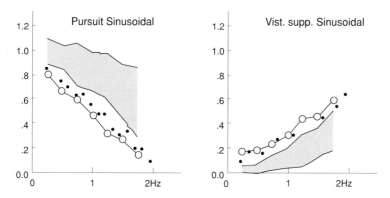

Fig. 3. Computerized smooth ocular pursuit with a pathologically low gain and pathological high gain in the visual suppression test in a patient with a cerebellar lesion. *Hatched area* indicates normative data; the *lines with the circles* are the recordings from the patient

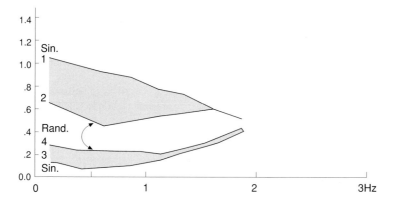

Fig 4. Smooth pursuit gain values for sinusoidal *(1)* and randomized *(2)* target movements in ten healthy volunteers. The *hatched area* indicates the difference between the results of the two tests. Visual suppression gain for sinusoidal *(3)* and randomized *(4)* rotatory stimulation is shown below with the same interpretation of the hatched area. (From [16])

70

Conclusion

In patients with balance disorders, vertigo, ataxia, or unilateral auditory problems there is a need for vestibular testing. On the basis of the case history and clinical examination the physician should be able to select the appropriate tests in the vestibular-oculomotor test battery. In ENG the caloric test will usually alert his attention to potential abnormalities. The test has the advantage that one ear at a time is investigated, but it is somewhat crude and not very specific. It should be pointed out that other electronystagmographic findings can be of greater diagnostic value: spontaneous nystagmus, gaze nystagmus, positional nystagmus or other abnormalities such as vertical nystagmus, pathological smooth pursuit or pathological visual suppression indicating CNS pathology. Rotatory testing is a more refined technique especially when it is performed with a broad frequency swing chair. This makes possible a comparison between the smooth pursuit function and the visual suppression mechanism, i.e. the visuo-vestibular interaction. Clinical investigation and posturography should also be included, and attention should be directed towards the influence of the neck on balance and oculomotor functions.

References

1. Ålund M, Ledin T, Ödkvist LM, Larsson SE, Möller C (1993) Dynamic posturography among patients with common neck disorders. A study of 15 cases with suspected cervical vertigo. J Vestibular Res 3:383-389
2. Aschan G (1966) Clinical vestibular examinations and their results. Acta Otolaryngol, Stockh [Suppl 224]:56-67
3. Bárány R (1907) Physiologie und Pathologie des Bogengang-Apparates beim Menschen. Deuticke, Vienna
4. Cramer RL, Dowd PJ, Helms DB (1963) Vestibular responses to oscillation about the yaw axis. Aerospace Med 34:1031-1034
5. Curthoys S, Halmagyi GM, Dai M (1991) The acute effects of unilateral vestibular neurectomy on sensory and motor tests of human otolithic function. Acta Otolaryngol, Stockh [Suppl 481]:5-10
6. Deblen J, Ledin T, Noaksson L, Ödkvist LM (1991) Visual suppression in the caloric and rotatory tests. In: Vertigo, Nausea, Tinnitus and Hypoacusea due to Head and Neck Trauma. In: Claussen CF, Kirtane MV (eds). International Congress Series 929, Elsevier, 25-29
7. Dichgans J, von Reutern GM, Römmelt V (1978) Impaired suppression of vestibular nystagmus by fixation in cerebellar and non-cerebellar patients. Arch Psychiatr Nerventer 226:183-199
8. Gripmark M, Ödkvist LM, Larsby B (1995) The subjective horizontal in eccentric rotation. Proceedings of the XXIth ordinary meeting of the Neorotologic and Equilibriometric Society, Hakone, Japan

9. Hydén D, Larsby B, Ödkvist LM (1983) Visual suppression tests in diagnosis of diseases of the central nervous system. Adv Oto-Rhino-Laryngol 30:205-209

10. Larsby B, Hydén D, Ödkvist LM (1984) Gain and phase characteristics of compensatory eye movements in light and darkness. A study with a broad frequency-band rotatory test. Acta Otolaryngol 97:223-232

11. Ledin T, Deblén J, Noaksson L, Ödkvist LM (1992) The head shaking test in the electronystagmography investigation. In: Claussen CF, KirtaneMV, Schneider D (eds). Conservative versus surgical treatment of sensorineural hearing loss, tinnitus, vertigo and nausea. Medicin + pharmacie, Dr Werner Rudat & Co, Nachf Edition, m+p, Hamburg

12. Möller C, Ödkvist L, White V, Cyr D (1990) The plasticity of compensatory eye movements in rotatory tests. I. The effect of alertness and eye closure. Acta Otolaryngol, Stockh, 109:15-24

13. Ödkvist LM (1988) Otoneurological diagnostics in posterior fossa lesions. Acta Otolaryngol, Stockh [Suppl 452]:12-15

14. Ödkvist LM (1988) Value of vestibular function tests in the differential diagnosis of vertigo. Acta Otolaryngol, Stockh [Suppl 460]:122-127

15. Ödkvist LM, Arlinger SD, Edling C, Larsby B, Bergholtz LM (1987) Audiological and vestibulo-oculomotor findings in workers exposed to solvents and jet fuel. Scand Audiol 16:75-81

16. Ödkvist LM, Thell J, Larsby B (1988) A comparison between smooth pursuit and visual suppression. Adv Oto-Rhino-Laryng 41:109-115

17. O'Leary DP, Davis LD, Kitsigianis GA (1989) Analysis of vestibulo-ocular reflex using sweep frequency active head movements. Adv Oto-Rhino-Laryn 41:179-183

18. Schwarz DWF, Tomlinson, RD (1979) Diagnostic precision in a new rotatory vestibular test. J Otolaryngol 8:554

PART 3

EVALUATION

Anamnesis and Clinical Evaluation

A. Cesarani, D. Alpini[1] and D. Brambilla[2]

Introduction

In all medical fields a good case history evaluation is the key to a correct diagnosis. Patients complaints have to be documented as completely as possibile from the beginning of the disease. Sometimes the examiner use of technical terms to question the patient can lead to confusion and misinterpretations. It is important that the patient describes symptoms with his/her own words in the simplest way. In this regard Grateu [3] proposed a simplified chart to investigate vertigo and dizziness during common daily life activities (Fig. 1). In whiplash equilibrium disturbances particular attention has to be paid to qualitative and quantitative aspects of symptomatology.

Qualitative Aspects

- Vertigo or dizziness: it is important to determine which is the prevalent symptom or if both are present or if there is a particular and recurrent sequence between vertigo and dizziness. For example dizziness appears when the patient removes the collar while performing normal activities, vertigo appearing during rotation or flexion-extension of the head.
- Onset of the symptoms: immediately after whiplash, or the day after, or when collar was removed, or when phisiotherapy began.
- Direction of vertigo rotation or the side of prevalent unsteadiness.
- Remission with particular position of the head/neck, generally the antalgic position.
- Combination with spinal pain and stiffness, brachial paresthesias, dysphagia or dysphasia, neurovegetative symptoms such as nausea and vom-

Ospedale Maggiore Policlinico, Istituto di Audiologia, Università degli Studi di Milano, Via Sforza 35, Milan, Italy
[1] ENT, Otoneurological Service Scientific Institute S. Maria N.te, F.ne don Gnocchi, Via Capecelatro 66, 20148 Milan, Italy
[2] IRCCS E. Medea, ᵃ Ass. La Nostra Famiglia, Otoneurologia, via Don Monza 20, Bosisio Parini (Co), Italy

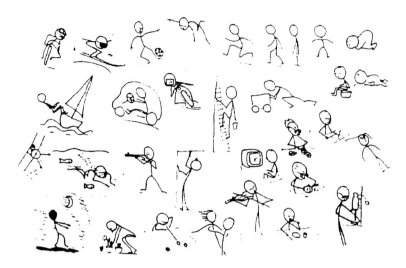

Fig. 1. Grateu's synoptic diagram for anamnesis

iting, cognitive symptoms such as amnesia and attentional disturbances, auditory symptoms such as hypoacusia and tinnitus.

- Loss of consciousness during whiplash, after it or combined with vertigo/dizziness.
- Headache and/or migraine immediately after the whiplash or in the following days/weeks/months.
- Incidence of symptoms on daily life activities. This qualitative aspect of symptomatology can be quantified using activities of daily life (ADL) questionnaires. As with functional scales, there is a tendency to use different standards, depending on the type of lesion one aims to study. However, the usefulness of questionnaires and ADL estimations should not be underestimated. The clinician may well use this information to enhance objective assessment of the patients. However, such estimations may be based and they can not easily be quantified or documented for studies or evaluation of the effect of treatment. To obtain better objective estimations several functional scales have been developed, generally designed for the study of a certain group of patients, thereby lacking the quality of general applicability. Well-known scales are the Tinetti subscale. A more generally applicable scale for patients with a disturbance in postural control is the balance scale suggested by Berg et al. [1], with a very easily applicable and redundant functional reach.

Quantitative Aspects

- Temporal distance between first medical visit and whiplash
- Temporal onset of each symptom and reciprocal combination
- Temporal relationship between symptoms remission or exacerbation and indemnity for personal damage
- Frequency of spontaneous attacks
- Intensity, quantified on a decimal scale
- Duration: continuous, subcontinuous, transient, recurrent.

Accident Aspects

- Whiplash of the driver or the passenger
- Anterior or posterior passenger
- Safety belts
- Rear-end or lateral or diagonal collision
- Collision with resting or moving car
- Position of the head during injury. For example if the passenger, with safety belt, was speaking with the driver with the car stopped for a traffic light, then a pure rear-end collisions would not induce a pure sagittal antero-retroflexion of the head but rather its torsional movement with the fulcrum on the first thoracic vertebrae and with a torsion of the trunk with the fulcrum on the first lumbar vertebrae. Such a complicated injuring mechanism usually induces a stronger longer lasting symptomatology, sometimes with severe vertigo and dizziness

In the medico-legal it field is very important to demonstrate the close correlation between trauma and patient complaints. In order to specify this relationship concomitant diseases and disorders have to be investigated:

- Vertigo or unsteadiness months or years before whiplash
- Previous trauma
- Previous otoneurological visit/ examinations either for symptoms or for working capability evaluation
- Previous auditory disorders
- Heart or brain or vascular diseases
- Hormonal disorders such as dysmenorrhea or dysthyroidism
- Metabolic disorders such as diabetes
- Use of alcohol, drugs, tobacco products
- Exposure to solvents or other cerebro-toxic factors
- Epilepsy
- Previous treatment for scoliosis or orthodontic problems which could influence postural system compensation possibilities
- Kinetosis.

During anamnesis, how the patient tells his own history can suggest to the clinician some other characteristics, such as anxiety, restlessness or depression. Sometimes specific psychometric scales can be used but they are generally not well accepted by the subject. Computerized anamnestic systems such as NODEC [2] are very useful in order to standardize the series of questions but reduce the interpersonal interaction between clinician and patient. Generally speaking we can say that computerized anamnestic systems are particularly indicated for those with medico-legal expertise, while personal anamnesis is more useful in treatment planning. The clinician has to identify psychological symptoms due to the stress of trauama and consequent symptoms or psychological habitus. During anamnesis the examiner may, if necessary, simply evaluate attentional disturbances with orienting (number of the present day), cultural (name of the Pope), memory (series of numbers), logic reversal ability.

Cerebellar coordination can be simply evaluated by asking the patient to provide his/her signature or draw a circle or a square. Visual-constructive functions can be investigated the Bender Gestalt visual-motor test. It is fast (15 min) and simple to perform for the clinician and for the patient. He/she has to copy as well as possible nine geometric paintings. The copies are then evaluated according to the Pascla-Suttel method (or Koppitz method for children 4-12 years). The aim of the test is to evaluate and quantify emotional disturbances.

Clinical Examination

As we said in the Introduction whiplash is a true non-contact cerebral trauma. Thus the neurootological and equilibrium examinations have to evaluate some neurological, orthopaedic and psychiatric aspects.

Cranial Nerves

Generally the olfactory nerve is not investigated routinely because it requires particular equipment (olfactometry). The opticus is clinically investigated evaluating the oculi fundus by means of an ophthalmoscope. Extrinsic and intrinsic ocular motility have to always be investigated. During oculomotoric extrinsic evaluation smooth pursuit and saccadic eye movements have to be investigated using a pen or the examiner's finger as target. Also the sensitivity of the face (trigeminus) and corneal reflexes has to be evaluated. Regarding the facial nerve for, mimic aspects are sometimes evident but dysesthesias of the auditory external meatus have to be searched for. The Shirmer test can complete the facial examination. Auditory function must be more

correctly investigated with the different audiometric tests leaving the diapa-
son tests to the history. Only the Weber test can be sometime useful during
clinical investigation. The inspection of the mouth and the larynx allows a
complete evaluation of cranial nerves IX, X, XII and eventually completed
with stimulation of the external auditory meatus and posterior pharyngeal
wall to induce, respectively, tussigenic and pharyngeal reflexes. The XI cranial nerve is usually evaluated during postural examination and palpation of
the sternocleidomastoidus and trapezius.

Posture Evaluation

Several approaches may be used to estimate human postural control and
they may be considered complementary. Clinical investigation can yield val-
uable information. Direct observation of the patient's behaviour, even during anamnesis, may contribute information otherwise overlooked. Several
generally well known examination procedures may be applied to help the
examiner evaluate the investigated subject. The use of standardized proto-
cols also gives the examiner more experience in interpreting the outcome of
the procedures. The active and passive movements of the head with respect
to the neck, the trunk and the pelvis must be estimated. Pain and movement
limitations have to be noted and in a certain way quantified. Palpations of
paravertebral extensory muscles, with special regard to those of the neck
and the back, have to be performed in order to appreciate hypo- or hypertonus of the muscles. Simple muscular force tests for the arm and leg extensors are useful. With the patient in a supine position a Babinsky test is simple
and informative. General muscular tonus can be simply evaluated by asking
the patient to resist with his/her thumb and index finger, contracting them in
a circle in response to an opposing force from the examiner.

Tendon reflexes may be simply investigated. Trigger and tender points
has to be routinely searched for along all paravertebral muscles and the tem-
poro-mandibular joint have to be inspected in static and dynamic (opening,
protrusion, laterotrusion) positions of the jaw.

During postural evaluation some sensorial evaluation can be contemporarily performed especially if paresthesias are complained of.

Vestibulo-spinal Examination

The classical Romberg test and the Fukuda and Unterberger stepping tests
are easily applied even in the office and may yield some information. A
patient unable to perform a Romberg's test will probably have prominent
difficulties in everyday life. During this test particular attention has to be

paid to the direction of the slow fall rather than the fast compensation. The Romberg test with feet in tandem position seems less appropriate as it requires a better than ordinary postural control and will yield a high degree of false-positive results. A Romberg's test with the neck extended, however, may contribute further information (Paulus, cited in [4]). In this position the lateral semicircular canal is brought into line with the gravity vector. A patient with a vestibular lesion causing ataxia and nystagmus falls in the direction of the slow phase of nystagmus while a patient with a cerebellar cause may fall toward the fast phase or the slow phase depending on the site of the lesion. According to Magnusson [4], the clinical headshake test and Romberg test may be performed at the same time. Nystagmus induced by a headshake test cannot differentiate between a CNS lesion or a peripheral vestibular lesion. One may, however, increase the sensitivity in tests of stance by combining the headshake test with a Romberg or a stepping test. The patient does headshakes for 10 s, standing with his back against a wall, then rapidly taking four steps forwards. If there is an evident deviation or fall toward the side of the fast phase of nystagmus induced by a previous headshake test, this may be taken as suggesting a posterior fossa lesion. Patients with compensated peripheral vestibular lesions seem to deviate only slightly. In whiplash injuries oculo-postural and neck-postural tests inform the examiner of the asymmetrical postural dynamic prevalence with special regard to cervical paravertebral muscles (for neck-postural). During stepping tests partuicular attention must be paid to coordination of movements, with special regard to the position and the stability of the head with respect to the neck.

Vestibulo-ocular Examination

Spontaneous nystagmusny has to be observed with and without fixation. Even if very often aspecific, spontaneous nystagmus is extremely sensible to every kind of vestibular impairment. Spontaneous nystagmus is the sole vestibular clinical and instrumental finding not voluntarily modifiable. In whiplash syndrome positional and positioning nystagmus and vertigo have to be always evaluated even if anamnesis is negative because positional, not always benign, vertigo is frequent. The head shaking test can not be always performed due to reduced cervical motility and pain. The qualitative and quantitative characteristics of spontaneous and positional nystagmus have to be noted with special regard to delay and fatiguability of positioning nystagmus. Furthermore it is important to note the temporal combination between nystagmus and vertigo: positioning or spontaneous vertigo without nystagmus; positioning or spontaneous nystagmus without vertigo; spontaneous or positioning vertigo and nystagmus. The influence of head position or changing the head position have to be researched in order to reveal the latent Moritz nystagmus.

Conclusions

At the end of a complete anamnesis and a complete clinical otoneurological examination the clinician has all the elements to plan the required instrumental tests. These can not substitute for the clinical sensitivity of the examiner but have to confirm, specify and document alterations of the equilibrium system. On the basis of anamnesis and clinical examination treatment planning can be generally completely performed even if instrumental tests are often indispensable to monitoring the results of therapy.

References

1. Berg KO, Maki BE, Williams JI, Holliday PJ, Wood-Dauphinee SL (1992) Clinical and laboratory measures of postural balance in an elderly population. Arch Phys Med Rehabil 73:1073-1080
2. Claussen CF (1992) Equilibriometric topodiagnosis as a basis of modern therapy of vertigo and dizziness. Neurootology Newsletter 1, 1:7-24
3. Grateau P (1992) Critique de l'objectivité? Neuromédia, Bull Club Neurosciences, 1986, DEA, Marseille
4. Magnusson M (1994) Evaluation of brainstem-cerebellar posture control. In: Cesarani A, Alpini D (eds). Equilibrium disorders. Brainstem and cerebellar pathology. Springer, Milan, 52-59

Voluntary Eye Movements in Whiplash Injuries

M. Spanio and S. Rigo

Saccades and smooth pursuit eye movements play an important role in the balance system. Essentially their aim is to free foveate animals from the slavery of oculomotor reflexes, such as vestibulo-ocular reflex (VOR) and optokinetic nystagmus (OKN). These voluntary eye movements enable the gaze to be rapidly redirected (saccades) or to slowly follow (smooth pursuit movements) new targets even when the head or surroundings are moving.

Saccades usually occur during VOR and OKN in order to automatically reset slow eye drift caused by vestibular or optokinetic stimuli and bring the gaze to the incoming scene, thus they have come to be known as nystagmus quick phases. Moreover saccades can help an oculomotor system which has been impaired by a pathology and override its resulting limitations. For instance, an abnormal smooth pursuit may present with saccades, seen on the eye record as a cog-wheel shape, which enhance global oculomotor response gain [1]. Even in labyrinth defective patients saccades represent a compensatory mechanism, taking on the role of the defective VOR [5].

The smooth pursuit system is perhaps involved in evoked nystagmus visual suppression, a function frequently investigated in clinical assessment of visual-vestibular interaction.

Therefore saccadic and smooth pursuit systems assist correct behaviour of the balance system, and, when affected by neurological lesions, they might lead to balance impairment, causing blurred vision and dizziness.

Saccadic and smooth pursuit are very complex oculomotor systems whose mechanisms have not yet been completely understood. As already stated the aim of a saccade is to quickly move the gaze onto a new visual target, therefore the stimulus consists in a gap between fovea and retinal target position, whereas the aim of a smooth pursuit movement is to follow a moving object, and here the stimulus consists in a velocity retinal slip between fovea and target.

The neural pathways of the two systems are completely different, but essentially they extend from cerebral cortex to brainstem oculomotor nuclei, passing through the cerebellum.

Clinica Otorinolaringoiatrica, Università di Trieste, Ospedale di Cattinara, 34100 Trieste (Italy), Tel. (39)-40-3994736, Fax (39)-40-3994793

Therefore abnormalities of saccades or smooth pursuit movements are considered a precise and sensitive marker of a central nervous system (CNS) pathology [7].

To record and analyse these ocular movements we require special investigative techniques and a well equipped laboratory.

In a clinical environment, visual stimulation is usually provided by a LED array and horizontal binocular movements are collected by means of DC-EOG and Ag-AgCl electrodes. As for the saccadic test, the subject is presented with predictable or unpredictable target jumps of several amplitudes (5°- 40°) in both directions (rightwards and leftwards).

As for smooth pursuit the subject is studied by using continuous target movements with triangular, sinusoidal or ramp patterns. Normally stimulus peak velocities of 20°- 40°/s are utilised.

Eye movements in saccadic tests are usually low-pass filtered at 50 Hz and sampled at 250 Hz, whereas data from smooth pursuit tests are low-pass filtered at 10 Hz and sampled at 50 Hz. Butterworth 18 dB/oct low-pass filters and 12-bit A/D conversion are used.

Analysis of saccadic movements is in two steps: first, a morphological evaluation of the global eye movement response to each target jump (overshoots, postsaccadic drifts, etc.); second, an automatic/interactive identification of the start and end points of each saccade, followed by an automatic evaluation of the saccadic parameters (latency, amplitude, duration and peak-velocity) for statistical analysis. Saccadic abnormalities are evaluated taking into account the direction and the amplitude of target displacement.

Analysis of the smooth pursuit responses is also in two steps: first, a morphological evaluation of the global eye response (both the smooth and saccadic components are investigated); second, evaluation of the gain and the temporal shift of the smooth component by cross-correlating the velocity of this component with that of the stimulus.

Although there is still debate as to its significance, a widespread clinical application of investigating the smooth pursuit system consists of a perrotatory nystagmus visual suppression test. The subject is rotated in darkness and asked to fix on a dim light rotating with him. With a healthy CNS the visual system can suppress perrotatory nystagmus down to 30% of the initial value or even lower.

In whiplash injuries it has been calculated that the sudden jerk of the neck can cause an elongation of the cervical columna up to 5 cm and thus an elongation of the brain stem [10]. This event can lead to, besides a wide range of lesions in the columna, nerve roots and medulla, even lesions in the brain stem, cerebellum and oculomotor system. Several authors have investigated the saccadic and smooth pursuit systems in whiplash patients.

Oosterveld et al. [8] submitted 262 patients, chronically suffering from the after-effects of whiplash, to an extensive vestibular and oculomotor ex-

84

amination. Some 85% of the patients complained of light-headness, spinning or floating sensations. Disturbances in visual pursuit movements were found in 113 patients (43%) and in visual suppression tests in 97 patients (37%), proving the presence of both cerebellar and brain stem pathology. However, a large number of patients (63%) also had a spontaneous nystagmus of more than 5°/s, interpreted by the Authors as a sign of central origin, which might interfere with smooth pursuit performance. In 41 patients oculomotor tests repeated 1 year later showed no significant improvements.

A high correlation between symptoms and oculomotor abnormalities has been found by Hildingsson et al. [2]. They examined the oculomotor function in 39 consecutive whiplash patients 6 months or more after the trauma. Twenty patients complained of chronic and disabling symptoms, such as neck ache, neck stiffness, headache, shoulder and arm pain. Two patients had vertigo or dizziness. Visual symptoms, often blurring of vision, as well as auditory symptoms were present in 15 patients. No difference in visual tracking was noted between 19 asymptomatic patients and control group subjects, whereas an oculomotor dysfunction was noted in 18 of 20 patients with persisting symptoms of a soft-tissue injury of the cervical spine. Four patients had pronounced abnormalities, and 14 had moderate oculomotor dysfunction.

In particular, smooth pursuit was abnormal with reduced velocity gain in 14 patients (in 12 asymmetrically) and with an increase in superimposed saccades in 16 patients (in 13 unilaterally). The saccades were hypometric in nine patients. Six patients had poorer accuracy and maximal velocity of the saccades, and five of these patients also showed latency prolongation. In general, patients with chronic symptoms had prolonged saccadic latency ($p < 0.001$).

Patients with more pronounced smooth pursuit abnormalities presented with saccadic dysfunction. None of the patients with saccadic dysfunction had normal pursuit.

The Authors suggest that the proprioceptive system in the cervicocranial area is affected in the 14 patients with moderate oculomotor impairment and that in the four patients with pronounced oculomotor abnormalities the brain stem and cerebellum are affected.

Successive observations of Hildingsson et al. [3] demonstrate that sometimes oculomotor systems disorders can occur at a later date. The AA investigated 40 consecutive whiplash patients. The most frequent acute symptoms after injury were aching and stiffness in the neck and headaches, followed by dizziness and shoulder pain. The initial oculomotor tests, performed within 3 months of the accident, were pathologic in eight patients. The follow-up test, on average 15 months after the accident, remained pathologic in the eight patients and a further five patients had changed from normal to pathologic test results. All the 13 patients with oculomotor dysfunction had disabling symptoms. In six patients smooth pursuit eye movements were abnormal with reduced velocity gain and with increased superimposed saccades. In all 13 patients the saccades showed low peak velocity and prolonged latencies. Three patients suffered pronounced abnormalities affecting both smooth pursuit and saccades.

Further support to the involvement of oculomotor systems in whiplash comes from the Odkvist et al. study [7]. The AA investigated 25 acute whiplash patients using, among other tests, smooth pursuit tests, saccadic tests and perrotatory nystagmus visual suppression tests. The patients were consecutive which meant that even lighter trauma could be included in the study. They were checked after 3, 6 and 9 months. At the first consultation about half of the patients had disturbances. The results are interpreted as indicating that pathological visual suppression and especially defective smooth pursuit ability may point to a chronic lesion of the brain stem. The patients concerned also had vertigo and unsteadiness. However there was no correlation between symptoms and pathological saccade tests.

Recently, in patients referred to our hospital for whiplash symptoms, we began a study of the VOR, and of a possible cervico-ocular component, by means of active and passive head movements. Out of these patients 14 were also submitted to saccade and smooth pursuit tests. The age of the patients ranged from 51 to 24 years (mean age 32.8 years); older patients were excluded in order to avoid impairment of saccadic and smooth pursuit performances due to aging or pathologies. Seven patients complained only of cervico-brachialgia or headache; seven complained also of dizziness and unsteadiness. All the patients were examined within a week of the accident. Even light trauma were included. The test results are reported in Table 1.

Saccade abnormalities appeared mostly in the symptomatic group, but even in some asymptomatic patients. A lower smooth pursuit gain was present only in symptomatic patients. The symptomatic group often presented a lower VOR gain. Only one asymptomatic patient presented a large phase lag of vertical VOR.

The number of patients examined is too small to draw a definite conclusion, nevertheless a relevant difference between our groups is the presence, in symptomatic patients, of an abnormality in at least one out of the three systems investigated. This might justify the balance disturbances the patients complained of. Nevertheless, the absence of a precise correlation between saccade abnormalities and symptoms, as found also by Ödkvist et al. [7], reduces the weight of saccade abnormalities on the balance. Even an isolated, but marked, saccade slowness cannot completely account for patients' complaints. Actually a low gain in the VOR or smooth pursuit has, on balance, greater effect than saccade slowness.

A summary of the above mentioned studies on whiplash injuries shows that saccade and smooth pursuit abnormalities are often present in symptomatic patients.

Table 1. Whiplash patients: oculomotor results

		Saccades			Smooth pursuit (gain)		VOR 1 Hz (gain/phase)	
	Main sequence	Latency	Metricity	Shape	20°/s	40°/s	Horiz.	Vert.
1	N	Increased	N	N	0.88	0.83	0.82/-5	1.05/-3
2	N	N	N	N	0.97	0.85	0.75/3	0.95/-5
3	N	N	N	N	0.98	0.80	0.73/-9	0.98/-6
4	PV ⇑ d ⇓	N	N	N	0.90	0.75	0.96/-6	0.91/-15
5	N	N	N	N	0.89	0.82	0.73/11	1.10/-11
6	N	N	N	Overshoots	0.97	0.87	0.75/-6	1.15/-13
7	N	N	N	N	0.90	0.82	0.80/2	1.15/-40
8	N	N	N	N	0.98	0.86	0.67/-5	0.65/-8
9	PV ⇑ d ⇓	Increased	N	N	0.99	0.68	1.07/-6	1.10/-10
10	N	N	Hypometria	N	0.94	0.62	0.93/-8	0.95/-13
11	PV ⇓	Increased	Hypometria	N	0.90	0.59	0.90/-2	0.89/-9
12	PV ⇓	N	N	N	0.78	0.65	0.65/-9	1.05/-10
13	N	N	N	N	0.85	0.78	0.69/-5	0.52/-10
14	PV ⇑ d ⇓	Increased	N	N	0.70	0.55	0.50/3	0.89/-4

PV = peach velocity; d = duration; N = normal parameters

If the impairments of saccades and smooth pursuit movements are considered a marker of a CNS pathology, how can their presence be explained in subjects affected by a soft tissue injury of the cervical spine, without assuming a contemporary head injury? Patients who received head trauma must have been excluded from data analysis. Therefore oculomotor abnormalities reveal damage of the CNS probably due to pull, stretch and pressure of the medulla oblongata, brain stem and cerebellum during the sudden jerk of the head [2, 3, 7, 8].

A different hypothesis has been proposed by Hinoki [4]. In patients with whiplash injury, there might be an overexcitation of the cervical and/or lumbar proprioceptors on the one hand, and a dysfunction of the CNS, such as the hypothalamus, the brain stem and the cerebellum, on the other hand.

These two factors cause imbalance by means of a trigger-and-target relationship in which the above proprioceptors act as a trigger and the CNS acts as a target. This hypothesis of a proprioceptive trigger, according to Hildingsson et al. [3], could explain even saccade and smooth pursuit abnormalities.

Nevertheless, a further element should be taken into account with regard to this type of oculomotor test. Saccades and smooth pursuit performances depend on cognitive functions to a large extent. Radanov et al. [9] evaluated the cognitive functions in whiplash patients and found they were impaired in terms of attention and speed of information processing.

These observations could justify some abnormalities: for instance latency increase in the saccades, and gain decrease in smooth pursuit movements.

In conclusion, the high incidence of saccades and smooth pursuit abnormalities in whiplash patients highlights the importance in investigation of whiplash injuries of oculomotor voluntary tests in order to prove the seriousness of the trauma. Nevertheless, these tests must be integrated into a larger clinical protocol aimed at the assessment of vestibular and optokinetic systems and postural control. Abnormalities in both saccadic and smooth pursuit systems may account for patients' complaints about balance only when the other tests provide normal results. The outcome of patient follow-up using these tests can be very useful both for patient control and medical-legal purposes.

References

1. Dell'Aquila T, Inchingolo P, Spanio M (1989) An analysis of the smooth and the global eye response to a periodic target motion in man. In: Schmid R, Zambarbieri D (eds). Proceeds Fifth European Congress on Eye Movements. University of Pavia, 76-78
2. Hildingsson C, Wenngren BI, Bring G, Toolanen G (1989) Oculomotor problems after cervical spine injury. Acta Orthop Scand 60 [5]:513-516
3. Hildingsson C, Wenngren BI, Toolanen G (1993) Eye motility dysfunction after soft-tissue injury of the cervical spine. A controlled, prospective study of 38 patients. Acta Orthop Scand 64[2]:129-132
4. Hinoki M (1985) Vertigo due to whiplash injury: a neurotological approach. Acta Otolaryngol, Stockh [Suppl 419]:9-29
5. Kasai T, Zee DS (1978) Eye-head coordination in labyrinthine-defective human beings. Brain Res 144:123-141
6. Leigh RJ, Zee DS (1991) The neurology of eye movements. Davis, Philadelphia
7. Ödkvist L, Alund M, Ledin T, Noaksson L, Deblen J, Moller C. Otoneurological disturbances in whiplash injuries (manuscript)
8. Oosterveld WJ, Kortschot HW, Kingma GC, de Jong AA, Saatci MR (1991) Electronystagmographic findings following cervical whiplash injuries. Acta Otolaryngol, Stock, 111:201-205
9. Radanov B, Dvorak J, Valach L (1992) Cognitive deficits in patients after soft tissue injury of the cervical spine. Spine 17[2]:127-131
10. Sances A, Weber RC, Larson SJ, Cusick JS, Myklebust JB, Walsh PR (1981) Bioengineering analysis of head and spine injuries. CRC Crit Rev Bioeng 6:79-122

Optokinetic Nistagmus and Visuo-vestibular Interaction in Whiplash Injuries

A. Salami, M. C. Medicina and M. Dellepiane

Introduction

The studies regarding cervical whiplash injury [12, 26, 28] showed that, in man, alterations can occur either in bands, muscles and neck vessels or - in very serious cases - in the CNS, cervical spine, brain stem, cerebellum, motor ocular system, as a consequence of the trauma [9, 15, 20, 36, 32], even without any bone lesions, which are seldom proved anyhow [22, 28]. These observations were confirmed by researches who showed the existence of various types of cerebral lesions (contusion, subdural hematoma and subarachnoidal or brain stem hemorrages) after cervical whiplash stress [30, 31].

Apart from the most serious neurological disturbances, otoneurological clinical features are very important elements in cervical whiplash. In particular, vertigo - which can be of different types - is one of the most common symptoms if not the most frequent one. Labyrinthic symptoms are variable in relation to either the type and intensity or the temporal course of clinical manifestations [22, 6, 32]. These symptoms include positional vertigo, which can also last for 2 years [8]; latent nystagmus which appeared in about 30% out of the patients either within or after a year following the trauma [43]; spontaneous nystagmus in more than 50% of the subjects, in most cases of positional type [32]. In many subjects the positional nystagmus was direction-fixed, in others direction-changing and the results of Dix-Hallpike manoeuvre suggested the possibility of otolithic damage with cupulolithiasis of the posterior semicircular canal [6]. We must also remember: the caloric tests' pathological results caused by lateral semicircular canal dysfunction [6], monolateral labyrinthic lesions in a certain number of subjects [32, 44]; a link with latent nystagmus, pathological monolateral caloric test and anomalous rotatory test, even later than a year after the trauma, in a great number of patients [44].

Oosterveld [32] and Ödkvist and coll. [29] also described alterations of the pursuit system and of the roto-acceleration nystagmus visual suppres-

Cattedra ORL, Ospedale Regionale S. Martino, Genova, Italy

sion test in patients who showed cerebellar and brain stem disease. Further observations, on patients with or without symptoms who were examined later than a year after the trauma, showed alterations either of pursuit system and saccades [15, 16] or of optokinetic nystagmus which are probably due to brain stem lesions.

On the basis of the reported data, which suggested the existence of complex peripherical and, overall, central alterations in the vestibular system as a consequence of a trauma in the cervical portion, we studied optokinetic and visual vestibular system behaviour in subjects who previously underwent a cervical whiplash injury; they often showed, even long after the date of the injury (expecially vertigo and headache) which were eventually liable to compensation.

The results of our research could be both interesting from a clinical point of view and useful for medico-legal goals. Our methods could be suitable for pointing out alterations in central sites as it is known that the nystagmus resulting from the contemporary optokinetic and roto-acceleration stimulation with counterdirectional nystagmus is significantly weakened in brain stem and cerebellar lesions and more widely in the presence of lesions in the posterior cranial fossa [33, 47, 38]. The visuo-vestibular interaction has not yet been adopted in the study of cervical whiplash injury.

Methods

The investigation was carried out on 32 subjects of age between 21 and 48 (18 men and 14 women) who had undergone a cervical trauma for a traffic accident with whiplash injury (Table 1). Thirteen subjects were examined within the third month following the accident (1st group), six subjects between the third and the sixth month (2nd group) and thirteen subjects later than 6 months up to 24 months (3rd group). It is important to note that we observed a spontaneous horizontal nystagmus in three subjects (one for each group) with an incidence of 9.3% out of the total.

Table 1. Complaints after cervical whiplash injuries in 32 patients

	Number	%
Headache	21	65.6
Subjective vertigo	13	40.6
Objective vertigo	4	12.5
Floating sensation	15	46.8
Tinnitus	14	43.7
Tinnitus and hearing impairment	5	15.6
Neck pain	13	40.6

The recording of ocular movements was done by the usual method using a Tonnies electronystagmograph with eight channels. The subjects were sitting with their heads still, on a Tonnies rotatory chair Pro model, which was placed in the middle of a rotatory cylindrical chamber with a diameter of 2 m and 1.9 m high. Its white internal area was covered with 32 black vertical contrasts (Fig. 1) each one 9.32 cm wide and with an angle of 5.61° [37]. The rotatory cylinder was lighted from above by a 100 Watt lamp and was driven by a direct current engine able to reach the desired turning speed (clockwise and counterclockwise) of up to 200°/s maximum speed, with preset acceleration ranging from 1°- 2°/s².

Each patient was exposed to: (1) *Postrotatory vestibular stimulation* (VOR, vestibular ocular reflex): with stop test, eyes open in the dark at an angular velocity of 90°/s which was subliminally reached clockwise and counterclockwise. (2) *Optokinetic stimulation* (OKN, optokinetic nystagmus) "stare type" with a cylinder rotation velocity of 30°/s for 60 s with clockwise and counterclockwise rotation. The lenght of 60 s was chosen because we thought that VOR could sometimes prevail over OKN. In this respect, our previous research on visuo-vestibular interaction [38-40] had shown that, in cases of lack of VOR substitution by OKN, sometimes it took more than 20 s for the appearance of OKN. (3) *Contemporary postrotatory vestibular and optokinetic stimulation* (VVOR, visuo-vestibular ocular reflex) at the post-rotato-

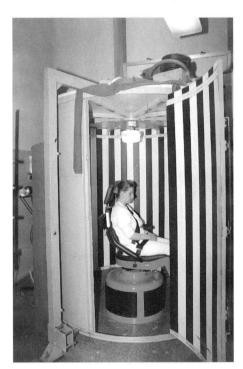

Fig. 1. Rotatory cylindrical chamber. The Tonnies rotatory chair system Pro in the middle

ry stop, the light was turned on and we effected optokinetic stimulation with a cylinder (and optical contrasts) rotation capable of inducing an OKN which was beating on the opposite side of the postrotatory vestibular nystagmus.

We took into account the fundamental parameter nystagmus "gain" as the ratio between the angular velocity of nystagmus slow phase and the stimulation velocity. VOR mean gain was calculated on the first three beats; OKN mean gain was calculated on the beats in the first 20 s; VVOR mean gain was calculated: (a) on the first three beats during the first 20 s of optokinetic stimulation, when the resulting nystagmus was beating in the OKN direction; (b) only on the first three beats, when the resulting nystagmus was beating in the VOR direction.

We used this method because, in VOR, there is a regular temporal decreasing phenomenon; OKN is - in relation to the length of our observation - a relatively constant phenomenon which does not show any signs of fatigue during the first 20 s [38, 39].

The results were compared with the ones we obtained in a group of seven normal subjects, ages 28-36, and statistically evaluated (mean difference) by t test.

Results

The results (Tables 2-4 and Figs. 2-5) can be summed up as follows:
VOR: none of the normal or pathological subjects showed any significant differences between the sides ($p > 0.05$). In pathological subjects mean gain decreased in all three groups compared with normal ones (Table 2) but it was statistically significant ($p < 0.05$) only in the subjects of the first group (Table 3), that is, in those subjets who underwent the trauma more recently.

Table 2. Mean with standard deviation of the mean gain

	VOR	OKN	VVOR OKN DIR [a]		VVOR VOR DIR [b]
	(3 beats)	(20 s)	(3 beats)	(20 s)	(3 beats)
Normal subjects	0.47±0.08	0.46±0.07	0.25±0.09	0.32±0.02	(–)
1st group (0-3 mos)	0.34±0.11	0.64±0.18	0.15±0.05	0.25±0.08	0.12±0.08
2nd group (3-6 mos)	0.45±0.12	0.73±0.09	0.22±0.14	0.29±0.19	0.18±0.13
3rd group (over 6 mos)	0.38±0.11	0.71±0.11	0.28±0.11	0.30±0.10	0.18±0.14

[a] OKN DIR, nystagmus beating in the OKN direction
[b] VOR DIR, nystagmus beating in the VOR direction

OKN: none of the normal or pathological subjects showed any significant differences between the sides ($p > 0.05$). In pathological subjects mean gain increased - with respect to normal ones - in all three groups (Table 2), with a significant increase ($p < 0.05$) in the first group and highly significant increase ($p < 0.01$) in the second and third groups (Table 3).

VVOR: in normal subjects VVOR always beats OKN direction, with a mean gain on the first three beats slightly inferior to the one calculated during the first 20 s (Table 2).

In 16 cases the pathological subjects' VVOR beat in the same direction of normal subjects (six in the first; four in the second; six in the third group) (Table 4), with a mean gain on the first three beats which only in the first group showed a statistically significant variation (decrease) ($p < 0.01$) compared with normal subjects (Table 3). In the three groups of pathological subjects the mean gain, during the first 20 s, showed a decrease compared to normal, but it was not statistically significant (Table 3).

In the remaining 16 cases (seven in the first; two in the second; seven in the third group) VVOR beat in the same direction as VOR (Table 4) for a variable length of 3 to 15 s (Figs. 3, 4) with a mean gain on the first three beats always highly inferior to VOR ones; VVOR beating in the VOR direction was followed by a variable period (a few seconds) of ocular immobility and then by a nystagmus beating in the OKN direction (Fig. 5).

Table 3. Significance test (*t*-test) between normal subjects and whiplash patients

	VOR (3 beats)	*ON* (20 s)	*VVOR OKN direction* (3 beats)	(20 s)
Normal vs 1st group	$p < 0.05$	$p < 0.05$	$p < 0.01$	$p > 0.05$
Normal vs 2nd group	$p > 0.05$	$p < 0.01$	$p > 0.05$	$p > 0.05$
Normal vs 3rd group	$p > 0.05$	$p < 0.01$	$p > 0.05$	$p > 0.05$

Table 4. VVOR in normal and in "whiplash" patients

	VVOR OKN direction	*VVOR VOR direction*
Normal	7	(–)
1st group (0-3 months)	6/13	7/13
2nd group (3-6 months)	4/6	2/6
3rd group (over 6 months)	6/13	7/13

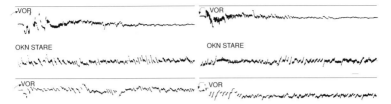

Fig. 2. Normal subject. *From top to bottom*: the postrotatory nystagmus (*VOR*) in the dark at the constant angular velocity of 90°/s with clockwise and counter clockwise chair rotation; optokinetic nystagmus "stare type" (*OKN*) with the cylinder rotatory constant velocity of 30°/s for 60 s; visuo-vestibular-ocular reflex (*VVOR*) with a cylinder rotation which caused an OKN beating on the opposite side of the postrotatory vestibular nystagmus. VVOR with counterdirectional VOR and OKN always evokes a nystagmus beating in the OKN direction

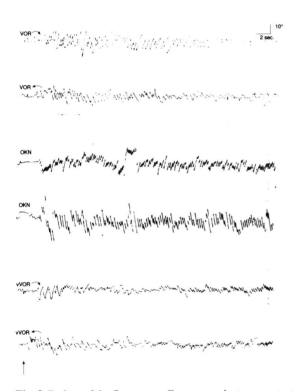

Fig. 3. Patient of the first group. *From top to bottom*: postrotatory nystagmus (*VOR*), optokinetic nystagmus "stare type" (*OKN* and visuo-vestibular-ocular reflex). Note: increase of OKN; VVOR is characterized by a nystagmus beating in the VOR direction for about 10 s. After a varying period of ocular immobility, a nystagmus beating in the OKN direction appeared. The *vertical arrows* point out the chair stop. For further information see Fig. 2

94

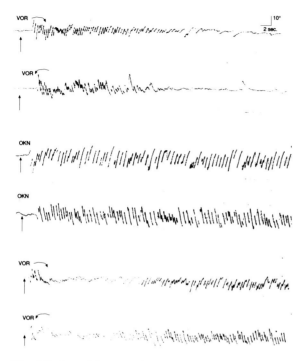

Fig. 4. Patient of the second group. We can observe a significant increase of OKN; VVOR is characterized by a nystagmus beating in the VOR direction for about 3 s. After a varying period of ocular immobility, a nystagmus beating in the OKN direction appeared. For further information see Figs. 2, 3

Discussion

The results of our research pointed to a statistically significant decrease of VOR and VVOR mean gains (beating in the OKN direction calculated on the first three beats) compared with normal subjects in the patients of the first group and a significant increase of OKN mean gain in the patients of all the three groups. Furthermore, at VVOR, immediatly after the stop, we observed a nystagmus beating in the VOR direction which lasted from 3-15 s in 16 patients out of 32 (seven in the first; two in the second; seven in the third group).

Miura [24] observed that cervical trauma of a certain extent (about 7 G) which was experimentally induced in rabbits, determined either microcirculatory alterations of brain stem and the superior portion of the spine or circulatory disturbances of the peripherical labyrinth. By analogy we can assume that the significant decrease of VOR mean gain that we observed in patients with cervical whiplash injury belonging to the first group could be

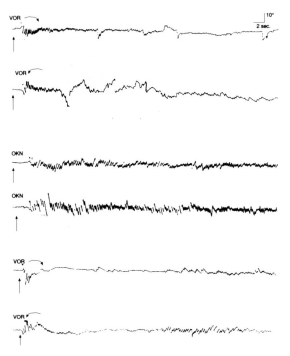

Fig. 5. Patients of the third group. We can observe an increase of OKN; VVOR is characterized by a nystagmus beating in the VOR direction for some seconds; after a varying period of ocular immobility, a nystagmus beating on the OKN direction appeared. For further information see Fig. 2

due to labyrinthic alterations subsequent to circulatory labyrinthic alterations. The possibility of damage, also minor, to peripheral vestibular structures as a direct consequence of cervical whiplash injury is also suggested by Chester [6] and by Brandt [4], as well as on the basis of the experimental data of Schuknecht and colleagues [41], who found a degeneration of Corti's organ and secondary of the pertaining acoustic fibers; these data could be taken into account in trying to explain, partially at least, the vestibular and audiological complaints (particularly hearing loss and tinnitus) referred to by some of our patients (Table 1).

As to the significant increase of OKN mean gain that we observed in all three groups, our results agree with those other Authors obtained [19, 18, 32]. If we take into account the importance either of vestibular nuclei in the production of OKN [45, 35] or of the pathway (even if it is not completely known) which is crossed by optokinetic impulses at the subcortical site (pretect and pontinus tegmen) [14, 3], and if we also consider that the cerebellar nodulus and flocculus receive visual and proprioceptive vestibular inputs

[42, 34, 5, 21], we may conclude that OKN increase in cervical whiplash injury is determined by: (a) pathological reactivity of vestibular nuclei caused by cervical propioceptors, i.e. "overexcitation" [17, 18], whose connections with brain stem and particularly with vestibular nuclei and reticular structure are already known [2, 11]; (b) an altered microcirculation of brain stem [25] and/ or by a neurological-vascular friction which may cause functional disorders of CNS and in particular of brain stem structures in cervical whiplash injury [18].

As to VVOR, it is known that the optokinetic-vestibular interaction with counterdirectional VOR and OKN evokes, in normal subjects, a nystagmus which is always beating in the OKN direction, with a mean gain decrease in relation to OKN [38, 39].

Our present results confirm these data as a further demonstration that a peripheral labyrinthic excitation, evoked by any technique and even if it is intense, induces, in normal subjects, a nystagmus which is always overcome by a contrasting OKN [7].

Nevertheless in six cases out of 13 patients belonging to the first group VVOR appeared with a nystagmus beating in the OKN direction, but with a mean gain - on the first three beats - which was significantly decreased compared with normal subjects. Finally in 16 out of 32 cases of the three groups (seven in the first; two in the second and seven in the third group) VVOR was characterized by a nystagmus beating in the VOR direction. These results recall some old observations by Cojazzi and Sala [7] and by Filippi [10], who observed a lack of substitution of caloric vestibular nystagmus caused by a contemporary optokinetic stimulation in cases of central vestibular alterations and in cases of monodirectional predominance of caloric nystagmus.

Numerous studies of animal anatomy and physiology showed the importance of the cerebellar flocculus in the working-out of visual vestibular interaction [1] and its influence on central velocity storage mechanism [27, 46, 13]. Therefore this structure is likely to be involved as a consequence of cervical whiplash injury, and an alteration may occur in the transmission of inputs coming from the caudal portion of inferior olive nucleus [40]. We may also face an alteration of the flocculus control function on vestibular inputs, as Miles and Fuller [23] have already showed.

From a clinical point of view these data confirm the importance of ENG examination in cervical whiplash injury. The alterations of OKN (statistically significant increase of mean gain in all three groups of patients) and of VVOR (nystagmus beating VOR direction) show - without reference to its pathogenetical origin - the presence of lesions, especially of central type and more specifically regarding brain stem and cerebellum. It is evident that these results are interesting from a medico-legal point of view. Therefore we can repeat Oosterveld and colleagues words: "In cases where legal medicine is involved, the outcome of an extensive nystagmographic examination can be of utmost importance both for the doctor and for the patients".

References

1. Baloh RW, Jenkins HA, Honrubia V, Yee RD, Law G.Y (1979) Visual-vestibular interaction and patients with cerebellar atrophy. Neurology, Minneapolis, 29:116
2. Boyle R, Pompeiano O (1981) Convergence and interaction of neck and macular vestibular imputs on vestibulospinal neurons. J Neurophysiol 45:852
3. Bon L, Corazza R., Iinchingolo P (1982) Oculomotor velocity efferent copy in the nucleus of the optic tract in the cat pretectum. Annual General Meeting of the European Brain and Behaviour Society, Parma
4. Brandt T (1984) Clinical evidence for cervical vertigo? In: Vertigo: its multisensory syndromes. Springer-Verlag, London 281
5. Carleton SC, Carpenter MB (1984) Distribution of primary vestibular fibers in the brainstem and cerebellum of the monkey. Brain Res 294:281
6. Chester JB (1991) Whiplash, postural control, and the inner ear. Spine 7:716
7. Cojazzi L, Sala O (1947) Sul diverso influsso del nistagmo otticocinetico sul nistagmo calorico in casi di iperreflessia vestibolare. Marginalia Otori-nolaryngologica 5:461
8. Compere WE (1966) Electronystagmographic findings in patients with "whiplash injuries". Laryngoscope 78:1226
9. Elliott F (1964) Clinical neurology. Saunders, Philadelphia
10. Filippo P (1949) Considerazioni sulla predominanza unidirezionale del nistagmo termico in alcuni casi otoneurologici. Arch Otol Rinol Laringol 60:235
11. Gacek RR (1982) The anatomical-physiological basis for vestibular function. In: Honrubia V, Brazier MAB (eds). Nystagmus and vertigo: clinical approaches to the patient with dizziness. AP, New York
12. Gay JR, Abbott K (1953) Common whiplash injuries of the neck. JAMA152:1698
13. Hasegawa T, Kato I, Harada K, Ikarashi T, Yoshida M, Koike Y (1994) The effect of uvulonodular lesions on horizontal optokinetic nystagmus and optokinetic after nystagmus in cats. Acta Otolaryngol Suppl 511:126
14. Henn V, Young L, Finley C (1974) Vestibular nucleus units in alert monkey are also influenced by moving visual fields. Brain Res 71:144
15. Hildingsson C, Wenngren B, Bring G, Toolenen G (1989) Oculomotor problems after cervical spine injury. Acta Orthop Scand 60:513
16. Hildingsson C, Wenngren B, Toolanen G (1993) Eye motility dysfunction after soft-tissue injury of the cervical spine. Acta Orthop Scand 64:129
17. Hinoki M (1972) Vertigo due to whiplash injury from the standpoint of neurootology. In: Itemi K (ed) Whiplash injury. Tokyo, Kanehara, Shuppan 100
18. Hinoki M (1985) Vertigo due to whisplash injury: a neurotological approach. Acta Otolaryngol, Stockh [Suppl 419]:9
19. Hinoki M, Hine S, Tada Y (1971) Neurotological studies on vertigo due to whiplash injury. Equil Res [Suppl 1]:5
20. Ikeda K, Kobayashi T (1967) Mechanisms and origin of so-called whiplash inury. Clin Surg 22:1655
21. Kano MS, Kano M, Maekawa K (1990) Receptive field organisation of climbing fiber afferents responding to optokinetic stimulation in the cerebellar nodulus and flocculus of the pigmented rabbit. Ex Brain Res 82:499
22. Jongkees LB (1993)Whiplash examination. Laryngoscope 93:113

98

23. Miles FA, Fuller JH (1974) Visual tracking and the primate flocculus. Science 189:1000

24. Miura Y (1968) Functional disorders of the blood vessels in the brain and spinal cord due to experimental whiplash injury. 27th Annual Meeting of the Jap Neurosurg Soc. Cited by Hinoki M (1985) Vertigo due whiplash injury: a neurotological approach. Acta Otolaringol, Stock [Suppl 419]:9

25. Miura Y, Tanaka M (1970) Disturbance of the venous system in the head and neck regions in rabbit with whiplash injury. Brain and nerve injury, Tokyo, 2:217

26. Mc Nab I (1982) Acceleration extension injuries of the cervical spine. The spine, vol II. WB Saunders, Philadelphia, 515

27. Nagao S (1983) Effects of vestibulocerebellar lesions upon dynamic charateristics and adaptation of vestibulo-ocular and optokinetic responses in pigmented rabbits. Exp Brain Res 53:498

28. Norris SH, Watti I (1983) The prognosis of neck injuries resulting from rear-end vehicle collision. J Bone and Joint Surg 65 B[5]:609

29. Odkvist L, Allund M, Ledin T, Noakssonn L, Deblen J, Moller C (1994) Otoneurological disturbances in whiplash injuries (manuscript)

30. Ommaya AK, Fass F, Yarnell P (1968) Whiplash injury and brain damage: an experimental study. JAMA 204:285

31. Ommaya AK, Hirsch AE (1971) Tolerances for cerebral concussion from head impact and whiplash in primates. J Biomech 4:13

32. Oosterveld WJ, Kortschot HW, Kingma GG, De Jong HAA, Saatci MR (1991) Electronystagmographic findings following cervical whiplash injuries. Acta Otolaryngol, Stockh, 111:201

33. Pfaltz CR, Bohmer A (1981) The influence of the pursuit and optokinetic system upon vestibular responses in man. Acta Oto-Laryng, Stockh, 91:515

34. Precht W, Volkind R, Maeda M, Giretti M (1976) The effects of stimulating the cerebellar nodulus in the cat on the response of vestibular neurons. Neuroscience 1:301

35. Precht W, Strata P (1980) On the pathway mediating optokinetic responses in vestibular nuclear neurons. Neuroscience 5:777

36. Rowe M, Carlson C (1980) Brain stem auditory evoked potentials in postconcussion dizziness. Arch Neurol 37:679

37. Salami A, Taborelli G (1984) Il nistagmo otticocinetico in camera ruotante. IV Giornata Italiana di Nistagmografia Clinica. Fisiopatologia del sistema vestibulo-visuo-oculomotore. Nistagmo otticocinetico. Movimenti di inseguimento. Movimenti saccadici. A cura di Dufour A, S. Vincent (AO)

38. Salami A, Filippi P, Mora E (1987) Il comportamento del nistagmo ottico-cinetico e del nistagmo d'interazione ottico-vestibolare nella patologia della fossa posteriore. VII Giornata Italiana di Nistagmografia Clinica. Terapia chirurgica della vertigine: indicazioni, limiti, prospettive. E.N.G. e patologia della fossa posteriore. A cura di Dufour A, Terme di Chianciano (SI)

39. Salami A, Bavazzano M, Tinelli E, Dellepiane M (1987) Il gain del nistagmo otticocinetico. Otorinolaringologia 37[2]:137

40. Salami A, Filippi P, Jankowska B (1988) Il comportamento del nistagmo ottico-cinetico e del nistagmo d'interazione ottico-vestibolare nella patologia degenerativa della fossa posteriore. VIII Giornata Italiana di Nistagmografia

Clinica. E.N.G. e patologia degenerativa tronco-cerebellare. Farmacologia sperimentale della vertigine. A cura di Dufour A, Montecatini Terme (PT)

41. Schuknecht HF, Neff WD, Perlman HB (1951) Experimental study of auditory damage following blows to the head. Ann Otol 60:273

42. Simpsom J, Alley K (1974) Visual climbing fiber input to rabbit vestibulo-cerebellum: a source of direction-specific information. Brain Res 82:302

43. Toglia JU (1976) Acute flexion-extension injury of the neck. Electronystagmographic study of 309 patients. Neurology 26:808

44. Toglia JU, Rosenberg PE, Ronis ML (1970) Posttraumatic dizziness. Vestibular, audiological and medicolegal aspects. Arch Otolaryngol 92:485

45. Waespe W, Henn V (1977) Neuronal activity in the vestibular nuclei of the alert monkey during vestibular and optokinetic stimulation. Exp Brain Res 27:523

46. Waespe W. Cohen B, Raphan T (1984) Dynamic modification of the vestibulo-ocular reflex by the nodulus and uvula. Science 228:199

47. Wennmo C, Hindfelt B, Pyykko I (1983) Eye movements in cerebellar and combined cerebello-brainstem diseases. Ann Otol Rhinol Laryngol 92:165

Vestibulo-ocular Reflexes and Visuo-vestibular Interaction

L. M. Ödkvist

Introduction

Human postural function uses afferent inflow from the inner ears, vision, pressure receptors in the soles of the feet, and proprioception in the extremities and back, especially the neck. Except for balancing and motor control the vestibular system plays a great role in ocular movements. The vestibular ocular reflex controlling eye movements is extremely quick and exact. The inner ear transduces the head movements and via the vestibulooculomotor reflex (VOR) the eyes are moved in such a way that the field of vision keeps steady on the retina. VOR is under the command of the central nervous system, especially the cerebellum and the prepontine reticular formation in the brain stem. The inflow from the neck plays an important role [11, 17, 22]. VOR elicits compensatory eye movements, i.e. the eye movements compensate for the head movements. The slow eye movement is regularly interrupted by a quick rebound phase and thus nystagmus appears with a slow and a fast phase. The slow phase has a speed of up to 60°/s, and the quick phase, the saccade, around 400°/s.

Animal experiments have shown the enormous inflow from neck muscle and ligament receptors to the vestibular nuclei in the brain stem. There is a large confluence of information via the inflow from inner ear, vision and proprioception on the nerve cells in the vestibular nuclei [16, 22]. Hence it is easy to realise the importance of the neck for the command of the movements of the body and balancing, as the inner ears only can report the position and movements of the head and not of the body. The vision registers the head position compared to the surroundings. Thus the neck has the important task of coordinating the proprioceptive inflow from extremities and back with visual and vestibular inflow.

Department of Otolaryngology, University Hospital, S-58185 Linköping, Sweden, Tel. (46)-13-222000, Fax (46)-13-222504

Examination

The vestibulo-oculomotor system can be approached in many ways. The *case history* is extremely important. The *clinical investigation* consists of ENT routine investigation, cranial nerves, balancing ability in the form of the Romberg test, cerebellar function investigation with, e.g. past pointing and diadochokinesis. The movements of the eyes are most easily investigated with the help of Frenzel glasses with 20 diopter lenses and inner illumination. One looks for spontaneous nystagmus, gaze nystagmus, positional and positioning nystagmus, neck torsion nystagmus and head shake nystagmus. The function of each inner ear is crudely tested with the help of the *caloric test*, irrigation of the ear canals with water 7°C above and below body temperature (hot and cold calorics). The result is a nystagmus for approximately 2 min, observed through Frenzel glasses.

For a more thorough investigation, *electronystagmography* (ENG) is necessary. ENG registers the movements of the eyes with the help of skin electrodes placed on each side of the eyes on the facial skin, horizontal and vertical to the eyes. The result after amplification is plotted on paper with the help of a computer presenting the results and simultaneously calculating the speed of the eye movements in the different parts of the investigation. The computer also calculates the result of the caloric test.

Important for the investigation of the influence of the central nervous system on eye movement is ocular smooth pursuit ability and quick eye movements, the saccades.

The *smooth pursuit test* uses a target moving over the field of vision with a known speed. ENG is recorded. The computer calculates gain, i.e. how exactly the eyes are pursuing the target [18, 23].

The *saccades test* uses alternatively light points, 10°, 20° or 30° apart. The gaze rests on one target a few seconds and then quickly moves over when the other target is lit. The computer calculates the latency, maximum speed, and accuracy of the saccade. Disturbances in the cerebellum and brain stem cause erroneous saccades [3, 23-25].

If the eyes gaze on a steady target while an inner ear stimulation is given, in the form of caloric irrigation or rotatory acceleration, a conflict appears between vision and VOR. The ability for vision and CNS to suppress the eye movements initiated in the vestibular system is called *visual suppression*, or cancellation of VOR, a function of the condition in the cerebellum and brain stem. With a healthy cerebellum the visual system can suppress VOR down to 30% of the initial value or lower. If vision is not able to manage this suppression it is called pathological, usually a sign of a lesion in the cerebellum or brain stem [7, 15, 18].

The real balancing ability is investigated with the Romberg test but is more accurately investigated with the computerized stance test - *dynamic*

102

posturography. The patient stands on a force-plate, coupled to a computer which registers and calculates the patient's sway during different conditions. The visual surrounding, a screen, is moved by the pressure of the feet on the computerized force-plate and thereby vision does not give much aid in balancing. Likewise the force-plate can be movable - sway referenced. By dynamic posturography the balancing ability can be calculated qualitatively and quantitatively [10].

For the investigation of patients with vertigo or balance disturbances, the function of adjoining *cranial nerves* is of importance especially the facial nerve and the auditory nerve. Modern *audiology* can very thoroughly decide the level of a hearing loss. As tinnitus often is a symptom when the neck is lesioned, hearing investigation is of uttermost importance.

Imaging in the form of X-ray computerized tomography (CT) and MRI (magnet resonance imaging) is sometimes necessary to find the lesion in the inner ear, the cranial nerves, the neck or the brain.

Vertigo Types

An *acute peripheral vestibular* loss is caused by, e.g. a fracture through the temporal bone and the inner ear or an inflammatory lesion of the vestibular nerve. It causes a nystagmus with a quick phase beating away from the side of the lesion - a destruction type of nystagmus. A slow central compensation appears day by day and week by week, faster in younger persons, slower in older patients.

A *slow loss* of function in an inner ear is rare but can be due to a tumour of the balance nerve causing the hearing gradually to disappear. The balance disturbance is usually compensated continuously.

A *fluctuating vertigo* can appear caused by a fissure from the inner ear after a trauma - inner ear fistula or membrane rupture. The symptoms can mimic those appearing in Menières disease. A fluctuating vertigo is common in connection with disturbances of blood pressure and cerebral circulation.

In rare cases vertigo can appear due to brain stem ischemia caused by compression of the vertebral artery when the head is turned. The artery passes through the foramina in the cervical vertebrae and from the first vertebra to the brain stem. Trauma or narrowing of the foramina can be the background to the ischemia according to this mechanism.

Neck Caused Vertigo

It has become more and more obvious that vertigo and balance disturbances can be caused by disturbances in tendons, joints and ligaments of the neck

[1, 2, 9, 12]. Lesions in the cervical roots and in the neck solid and soft tissues can disturb vestibulo-oculomotor functions. The vestibular nuclei in the brain stem and the cerebellum receive afferent projections from the cervical dorsal roots. These connections are dominated by muscle afferents. Hence a vestibular disturbance is possible with tension and pain of the neck muscles. Adjoining symptoms may be movement pain or pain at rest in the neck, tender muscles, headache and decreased mobility in the neck. The afferent nervous inflow is misinterpreted by the brain stem as movement, and thus the oculomotor system reponds with nystagmus.

The investigation may also show that there is hyper- and hypomobility in different segments of the cervical column, diminished ability to turn, flex or extend the cervical column. Treatment with physiotherapy, acupuncture or other methods can often successfully cure the pain and the headache as well as the vertigo [14, 19]. When the patient returns to the doctor after physiotherapy and/or acupuncture and the neck pain is gone simultaneously with the disappearance of vertigo, the connection between the neck disturbance and vertigo becomes clinically obvious [1].

Whiplash and Vestibulo-oculomotor Disturbances

When a person is sitting in a car which is hit from the rear, the head is caught by the neck support in the first movement and later thrown forward. The thorax is caught by the safety belt. The force acting on the head in the anterior direction has been calculated to possibly reach 12 G, an enormous power. The whole event takes about 20 ms but the reaction time for the muscles is 50 ms. Obviously they do not have time to react and protect the head and the neck for the extension that is created. It has been calculated that this sudden jerk in the neck can cause an elongation of the cervical columna as much as 5 cm [21]. Three types of disturbances may appear: lesions of the temporal bone and the inner ear, lesions of the neck proprioceptive system, and due to the elongation of the cervical spine also disturbances of the structures in the posterior cranial fossa, i.e. the cerebellum and brain stem. All these types of lesions may have implications on the funtion of the oculomotor system [2, 6, 8, 13, 14, 21, 20].

In the Netherlands, Oosterveld et al. [21] investigated 262 patients, 5 months to 5 years after traffic accidents with whiplash trauma, suffering from the late results of the whiplash lesion. The patients came to the investigation due to headache, neck pain, vertigo, unsteadiness, tinnitus or disturbed brachial sensation. The symptoms had been present for more than 4 months. Among the patients there were also frequent complaints of concentration difficulties and disturbances of memory as well as vertigo and some visual problems. Spontaneous nystagmus was present in 63% of the cases, neck torsion nystagmus in 79%, disturbances of visual suppression in 37% and disturbances of the ocular pursuit ability in 43%. Oosterveld et al. interpreted this as brain stem and cerebellar lesions and stressed the importance of ENG for a complete investigation of whiplash patients.

Hinoki [6], in a Japanese study, pointed out several different mechanisms for disturbances after a whiplash lesion: overexcitation of the cervical proprioceptors, sympathetic system disturbances and also lesions in the cerebellum and brain stem.

In Sweden, Hildingsson et al. [4, 5], in two studies, have investigated whiplash patients. In 20 patients with disturbances at least 1 year after whiplash violence, neck symptoms were present and in 18 patients vertigo in some form. Blurred vision and tinnitus were present in 15 patients. Of the patients with symptoms 14 had disturbed smooth pursuit ability and nine had pathological saccades. A control group and a group with neck trauma but without symptoms had normal findings in the oculomotor tests. In the second study with 40 consecutive cases of whiplash violence, 13 patients at follow-up had pathology in the oculomotor tests. Five patients had symptoms disturbing the working ability but had normal eye movements. Five others had pathological eye movements, although they had been normal at the initial investigation. The conclusion is that smooth pursuit tests and saccade ability were disturbed due to brain stem lesions in whiplash patients.

Our study in 25 patients who came for acute consultation after whiplash trauma in traffic accidents were investigated after 1 week, 3 months, 6 months and 9 months [20]. The cases were consecutive which meant that even lighter trauma patients were included in the study. The investigation included auditory tests, ENG, computerized smooth pursuit test, computerized saccade test, rotatory test with visual suppression and dynamic posturography. At the first consultation about half of the patients had positive findings. Our interpretation is that the patients have a chronic lesion of the brain stem causing pathological visual suppression and, even more, a pathological ocular smooth pursuit ability. These patients also had vertigo and unsteadiness. In our study there was not the same obvious correlation between symptoms and pathological saccades as in the Hildingsson study [4, 5]. There even appeared pathological dynamic posturography but the correlation was not as obvious as in our earlier study with dynamic posturography in 25 patients with typical cervical vertigo [1].

Conclusions

Vertigo and balance disorders may, for different reasons, appear as a result of a whiplash injury. One reason may be a lesion in the muscles, joints and ligaments of the neck causing cervical vertigo for a shorter or longer period of time. Vertigo and balance disturbances may even appear due to a brain stem lesion or a cerebellar lesion appearing at the moment of trauma due to an elongation of the brain stem, when the head, with great power, is pulled forward [21]. The pathological findings may be more difficult to interpret if, due to a trauma to the ear with an inner ear concussion or fistula or a simultaneous temporal bone fracture, there is an inner ear lesion with vertigo and disturbed balance. Also traumatic brain or cerebellar damage has to be taken into consideration. Oculomotor testing with ENG is mandatory for diagnostic, prognostic and legal purposes.

Except for neck investigation the patients with cervical vertigo and whiplash injury must be investigated concerning hearing, balance and eye movements. This is performed by clinical investigation, audiometry, posturography and ENG. Testing of saccades, smooth pursuit and visual suppression calls for special investigation techniques in a well equipped laboratory.

References

1. Ålund M, Ledin T, Ödkvist LM, Larsson S-E, Möller C (1993) Dynamic posturography among patients with common neck disorders. A study of 15 cases with suspected cervical vertigo. J Vestibular Res 3:383-389
2. Depondt M (1974) Le nystagmus d'origine cervicale. Acta Otorhinolaryng, Belg 28:759
3. Henriksson NG, Hindfelt B, Pyykkö I, Schalén L (1981) Rapid eye movements reflecting neurological disorders. Clin Otolaryngol 6(2):111-119
4. Hildingsson C, Wenngren BI, Bring G, Toolanen G (1989) Oculomotor problems after cervical spine injury. Acta Orthop Scand 60:513-516
5. Hildingsson C, Wenngren BI, Toolanen G (1993) Eye motility dysfunction after soft-tissue injury of the cervical spine. Acta Orthop Scand 64(2):129-132
6. Hinoki M (1985) Vertigo due to whiplash injury: a neurotological approach. Acta Otolaryngol, Stockh [Suppl 419]:9-29
7. Hydén D, Larsby B, Ödkvist LM (1984) Quantification of compensatory eye movements in light and darkness. Acta Otolaryngol, Stockh [Suppl 406]:209-211
8. Ikeda K, Kobayashi T (1967) Mechanisms and origin of so-called whiplash injury. Clin Surg 22:1655-1660
9. Jongkees LB (1969) Cervical vertigo. Laryngoscope 79:1473
10. Ledin T, Ödkvist LM, Vrethem M, Möller CG (1991) Dynamic posturography in assessment of polyneuropathic disease. J Vest Res 1:123-128
11. Liedgren SRC, Rubin AM, Aschan G, Ödkvist LM, Larsby B (1978) Influence of neck afferents on activity in the cat vestibular nuclei. In: Hood JD (eds). Vestibular mechanisms in health and disease. Academic Press, London 8:18-27
12. Liedgren SRC, Ödkvist L (1979) The morphological basis for vertigo of cervical orgin. Proc Neurootol Equilibr Soc, pp 153-165
13. Macnab I (1971) The "whiplash syndrome". Orthop Clin North Am 2(2):389-403

14. Norris S H, Watt I (1983) The prognosis of neck injuries resulting from rear end vehicle collisions. J Bone Joint surg (Br) 65(5):608-611
15. Ödkvist LM (1988) Otoneurological diagnostics in posterior fossa lesions. Acta Otolaryngol, Stockh [Suppl 452]:12-15
16. Ödkvist LM, Larsby B, Fredrickson JM (1975) Projection of the vestibular nerve to the SI arm field in the cerebral cortex of the cat. Acta Otolaryngol, Stockh, 79:88-95
17. Ödkvist LM, Liedgren SRC, Larsby B, Jerlvall L (1975) Vestibular and somatosensory inflow to the vestibular projection area in the postcruciate dimple region of the cat cerebral cortex. Exp Brain Res 22:185
18. Ödkvist LM, Thell J, Larsby B (1988) A comparison between smooth pursuit and visual suppression. Adv Oto-Rhino-Laryngol 41:109-115
19. Ödkvist I, Ödkvist LM (1988) Physiotherapy in vertigo. Acta Otolaryngol, Stockh [Suppl 455]:74-76
20. Ödkvist LM, Ålund M, Ledin T, Noaksson L, Möller C (1995) The role of posturography and electronystagmography in whiplash injuries. In: Proceedings of the XXIth ordinary meeting with the Neurotological and Equilibriometric Society, Hakone, Japan
21. Oosterveld WJ, Kortschot HW, Kingma G, de Jong HAA, Saatci MR (1991) Electronystagmographic findings following cervical whiplash injuries. Acta Otolaryngol, Stockh, 111:201-205
22. Rubin A, Liedgren SRC, Ödkvist LM, Milne AC, Fredrickson JM (1978) Labyrinthine and somatosensory convergence upon vestibulo-ocular units. Acta Otolaryngol, Stockh, 85:54-62
23. Schalén L, Henriksson N G, Pyykkö I (1982) Quantification of tracking eye movements in patients with neurological disorders. Acta Otolaryngol, Stockh, 93(5-6):387-395
24. Wennmo C, Hindfelt B (1980) Eye movements in brainstem lesions. Acta Otolaryngol, Stockh, 90(3-4):230-236
25. Wennmo C, Hindfelt B, Pyykkö I (1983) Eye movements in cerebellar and combined cerebello-brainstem diseases. Ann Otol Rhinol Laryngol 92(2):165-171

Abducting Interocular Ophthalmoplegia After Whiplash Injuries

D. Alpini, A. Cesarani[1] and E. Merlo[1]

Introduction

Internuclear ophthalmoplegia (INO) is a well recognizable disorder of horizontal eye movements and it is a common finding in neurological disorders [15].

INO is due to a functional impairment of the medial longitudinal fascicle (MLF) ipsislateral to the medial rectus paresis. Generally INO is characterised by the impairement of adduction of the eye on the side of the impaired MLF and abduction overshoot. The electro-oculographic saccadic and gaze nystagmus patterns are typical.

In whiplash injuries ocularmotor disturbances are frequent also in those patients in whom a head trauma did not occur [8, 10, 18]. In rare cases [1] eye movement disorders are characterised by ocular conjugate movement impairment sometimes as typical INO, sometimes as isolated abducens palsy.

With a certain frequency we observed "atypical" abducting ophthalmoplegia pattern, characterised by bilateral impairment of the velocity of the abducting eye [3, 5, 6].

This finding was described by Lutz [14], who proposed the existence of an abduction paresis of prenuclear origin (ophthalmoplegia internuclearis posterior, pINO). As his basic neuroanatomical assumptions were erroneous, the existence of this kind of INO remained controversial and papers in the literature are quite rare.

Abduction INO differs from abducens nerve palsy in several aspects, such as absence of strabismus and diplopia in the primary position and adduction nystagmus of the contralateral eye [11-13].

The aim of this chapter is to report the frequency of abducting INO that occurred in a group of patients after whiplash injuries without head trauma and to discuss possible etiopathogenic mechanisms.

ENT, Otoneurological Service Scientific Institute S. Maria N.te, F.ne don Gnocchi, Via Capecelatro 66, 20148 Milan, Italy
[1] Ospedale Maggiore Policlinico, Istituto di Audiologia, Università degli Studi di Milano, Via Sforza 35, Milan, Italy

Material and Methods

Twentythree consecutive subjects were investigated: 16 women and seven men with mean ages of, respectively, 31.35 and 34.7 years (from 16 to 70 years).

Eye movements were recorded in DC by a computerized Nicolet Biomedical Nystar electro-oculograph, using monocular electrodes. Eye movements were elicited by the mean of a semicircular LED bar and the following tests were performed:
- Horizontal and vertical random saccades from 6° to 32°
- Sinusoidal 0.2 and 0.4 Hz horizontal smooth pursuit and 0.2 vertical smooth pursuit
- 40°/s bidirectional horizontal OKN and 20°/s vertical OKN

The following paramethers were calculated:
- Saccades: delay, accuracy, number, performance index, mean velocity at each amplitude
- Smooth pursuit: gain, DC offset, total harmonic distortion, maximum velocity - OKN: number of beats; frequency; maximum velocity; gain
- Sinusoidal provoked nystagmus (0.5 Hz at 11.5 and 5.75°/s^2) in the dark (VOR) and in the light (VVOR): nystagmus frequency and mean slow phase velocity (SPV) and VVOR gain (VVOR-SPV/VOR-SPV).

Results

The presence of bilateral abducting eye slowing was evaluated comparing accuracy, performance index and saccadic eye velocity with the normal values previously calculated in a group of 25 normal adults. No patients showed slowing of the adducting eye or another pattern like typical INO.

Horizontal saccades revealed slowing of the abducting eye in eight patients (ABD) (34.7%): two men and six women with mean ages of 35.87

Table 1. Percentages of pathological tests in patients with (ABD) and without (no-ABD) abducting interocular ophthalmoplegia

	ABD	no-ABD
Horizontal saccades	62.5%	20%
Vertical saccades	25%	26.6%
Horizontal smooth pursuit	37.5%	40%
Vertical smooth pursuit	25%	33.3%
Horizontal OKN	25%	20%
Vertical OKN	0%	6.6%
VOR	37.5%	40%
VVOR gain	25%	66.6%

years (from 16 to 58 years). The mean age of the group of patients without abducting slowing was 33.67 years (from 19 to 70 years).

In Table 1 the distribution of altered neurotological tests is shown. The percentages of altered tests regarding patients with abducting eye slowing are referred to alterations of parameters other than eye velocities, such as latency, accuracy, offset, directional preponderance.

Horizontal saccades are altered in 62.5% of ABD patients versus 20% of the other group. All the other ocularmotor tests are altered in the same manner in the two groups of patients (with exception of VVOR).

Discussion

Internuclear ophthalmoplegia can be attributed to a lesion of the MLF between the levels of the third and sixth nucleus [7, 9, 16]. It has been assumed that the lesion affects axons arising from cells in the paramedian pontine reticular formation (PPRF) but this is not an accepted explanation for every cases. In fact the impairment of movement is variable, the most severe lesions causing complete loss of adduction beyond the midline during contralateral gaze; in some cases the impairment also affects the convergence mechanism while in others convergence is normal.

Cogan [4] divided INO into anterior and posterior types according to whether the convergence was normal or not, while Lutz [14] divided INO into anterior and posterior according to whether the medial or the lateral rectus muscle was paralysed. If convergence is still possible it seems to be difficult to distinguish monolateral INO of abduction from abducens paralysis while bilateral abducting INO may refer only to a lesion of the internuclear fibres.

There has been little agreement on the location of the responsible lesion and the pathophysiological explanation of abducting INO. Some authors [2, 3, 5], rejecting the existence of a prenuclear abduction paresis, attributed such cases to the pontine involving the abducens nerve along its infranuclear intrapontine course. Others [17, 18, 19] postulated decreased excitation of the lateral rectus motor neurons due to a lesion of prenuclear structures, that is, aberrant "pyramidal tract" fibres to the abducens nucleus or the connection between the PPRF and the ipsilateral abducens nucleus. An impaired inhibition of the antagonistic medial rectus muscle was discussed by Collard et al. [5] suggesting a MLF lesion contralateral to the paretic eye.

Thomke et al. [19] demonstrated that the lesion is ipsilateral to the abduction paresis at the upper pons or midbrain level. They also showed the existence of a fasciculus near the MLF specific for inhibition of medial rectus. They stated that ABD ophthalmoplegia is due to impaired inhibition of medial rectus tonic resting activity following interruption of this para-MLF fasciculus.

In our opinion, despite the controvers about the physiopathology of abducting ophthalmoplegia, the term of "abducting *interocular* ophthalmoplegia" is preferable rather than the classical "internuclear". In our experience this pattern is not rare and, if monocular ENG recording is routinely performed, it describes a third of the patients suffering vertigo and or dizziness after whiplash injuries, even without minor or major head trauma.

In Fig. 1 a case of abducting interocular ophthalmoplegia following whiplash is showed. The involved parameters are peak velocities/ movement amplitude ratio (the butterfly diagram) and the percentages of accuracy, comparing abducting and adducting movements.

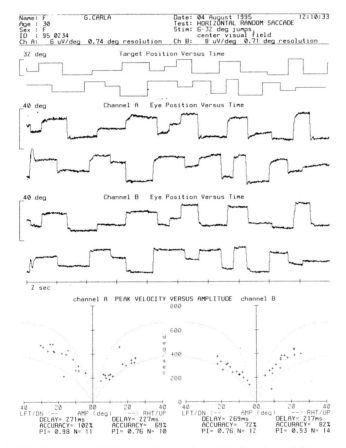

Fig. 1. A case of abducting interocular ophthalmoplegia following whiplash. The involved paramethers are peak velocities/ movement amplitude ratio (the *butterfly diagram*) and the percentages of accuracy, comparing abducting and adducting movements. The *PI* (performance index) refers to patient peak velocities compared to normal values previously stored in the program

The PI (performance index) refers to patient peak velocities compared to normal values previously stored in the program.

It is interesting to reveal that neuro-otological differences in the two groups of patients concerns, in an opposite way, horizontal saccades and VVOR.

In fact in the ABD group horizontal latencies or adducting accuracies (parameters different from those correlated to abducting eye slowing) were altered in 62.5% versus 20% of the other subjects, while VVOR was normal in 75% and altered in 66.6% of no-ABD patients.

In no case was *adducting* slowing recorded and we know only one paper in the literature describing INO after whiplash without head trauma [10].

If we hypothesize a brain stem lesion with para-MLF involvement due to neck hyperextension there will be no need to exclude the possibility of the neurologically most frequently occurring adducting ophthalmoplegia. Our cases are not misdiagnosed bilateral abducens palsy as described [18] either on the basis of the clinical considerations reported in the Introduction or on the basis of ophthalmological examination excluding abducens palsy.

In our opinion abducting interocular ophthalmoplegia has to be considered a disorder of ocular coordination correlated to head/neck and head/eye coordination disorders caused by whiplash. It must not necessarily be correlated to a brainstem lesion.

References

1. Baker RS, Epstein ADD (1991) Ocular motor abnormalities from head trauma. Surv Ophthalmol 35:245-267
2. Bakheit AM, Behan PO, Melville ID (1991) Bilateral internuclear- ophthalmoplegia as a false localizing sign. J R Soc Med, England 84:627-630
3. Bronstein AM, Rudge P, Gresty MA, Boulay G, Morris J (1990) Abnormalities of horizontal gaze. Clinical, oculographic and magnetic resonance imaging findings. II. Gaze palsy and internuclear ophthalmoplegia. J Neurol Neurosurg Psychiatry 53:200-207
4. Cogan DG, Kubik CS, Smith WL (1950) Unilateral internuclear ophthalmoplegia; report of eight clinical cases with one postmortem study. Arch Ophtalm 44:783
5. Collard M, Eber AM, Streicher D, Rohmer F (1979) L'ophtalmoplegie internucleaire posterieure-existe-t-elle? A propos de onze observations avec oculographie. Rev Neurol 135:293-312
6. De Keizer RJW, Zee DS (1987) Eye movement disorders. In: Sanders EACM, De Keizer RJW, Zee DS (eds). Martinus Nijhoff, Dr W Junk, Dordrecht, 186
7. Haller KA, Miller-Meeks M, Kardon R (1990) Early magnetic resonance imaging in acute traumatic internuclearophthalmoplegia. Ophthalmology 97:1162-1171
8. Hildingsson C, Wenngren BI, Bring G, Toolen G (1989) Oculomotor problems after cervical spine injury. Acta Orthop Scand, Denmark, 60:513-516
9. Hopf HC, Thomke F, Gutman L (1991) Midbrain vs. pontine medial longitudinal fasciculus lesions: the utilization of masseter and blink reflexes. Muscle Nerve

14:326-330
10. Jammes JL (1989) Bilateral internuclear ophthalmoplegia due to acute cervical hyperextension without head trauma. J Clin Neuro Ophthalmol 9:112-115
11. Kommerell G (1975) Internuclear ophtalmoplegia of abduction. Arch Opthalmol 93:971-980
12. Larmande AM (1969) La paralysie supranucleaire du VI (dite ophtalmoplegie internucleaire posterieure). Arch d'Ophtalmol, Paris, 29:521-530
13. Lee J, Flynn JT (1985) Bilateral superior oblique palsies. Br J Ophthalmol 69:508-513
14. Lutz A (1923) Ueber die Bahnen der Blickwendung und deren Dissocierung. In: Sanders EACM (ed). Syndromes of the medial longitudinal fasciculus. Klin Monatsbl Augenh 70:213-235
15. Oosterveld WJ, Kortschot HW, Kingma GG, de Jong HA, Saatci MR (1991) Electronystagmographic findings following cervical whiplash injuries. Acta Otolaryngol, Stockh, 111:201-205
16. Sanders EACM, De Keizer RJW, Zee DS (1987) Eye movement disorders. Martinus Nijhoff, Dr W Junk, Dordrecht
17. Sanders EACM (1987) Syndromes of the medial longitudinal fasciculus. In: Sanders EACM, De Keizer RJW, Zee DS (eds). Eye movement disorders. Martinus Nijhoff, Dr W Junk, Dordrecht, 183
18. Shifrin LZ (1991) Bilateral abducens nerve palsy after cervical spine extension injury. A case report. Spine 16:374-375
19. Thomke F, Hopf HC, Kramer G (1992) Internuclear ophthalmoplegia of abduction: clinical and electrophysiological data on the existence of an abduction paresis of prenuclear origin. J Neurol Neurosurg Psychiatry 55:105-111

Instrumental Evaluation of the Posture

M. MAGNUSSON

Introduction

Most common human activities require the ability to stabilize the human body in upright stance, to counteract perturbations and to allow voluntary movements, according to gravitational forces. The standing human is an unstable physical structure. To counteract the effects of gravity and comply with the requirements to stabilize the body during voluntary movements there is a continuous modulation of motor activity, especially in so-called anti-gravity muscles, based on the also continuously changing afferent sensory information (Fig. 1). The postural control of the standing human can therefore be considered in part a dynamic feedback control [1]. Furthermore, based on experience and visual information, the standing human may foresee per-turbations or changing requirements in advance, thus adding a substantial degree of anticipatory or feed-forward control [2]. To evaluate the signifi-cance on postural control of observations or test results it is necessary to bear in mind the physiological background and ability to maintain upright stance. Postural control cannot be considered a strictly hierarchical system but rather is characterized by decentralized or local decisions in a way which allows comparisons with the popular algorithms of neural networks [2]. Fur-thermore, there is a substantial amount of redundancy [2, 3]. The comple-mentary relationships between the afferent orientational information, i.e. the visual vestibular and somatosensory information, in postural control has been well known since the observations of Romberg in the nineteeth century. However, the redundancies of the sensory systems or the central nervous pathways should not be interpreted as the information from the different sensory systems or neural pathways being equivalent and interchangable. Instead there is evidence emerging which suggests that in cases of lesions or loss of information from one receptor or control system, another set of com-mands or strategy may be used to regain a sufficient postural control [4]. If so, there should be possibilities to evaluate the effects and differences of various lesions and the applied therapies.

Department of Otorhinolaryngology, University Hospital, Lund, Sweden

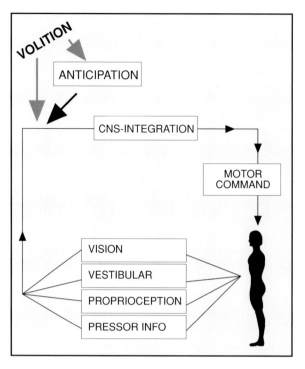

Fig. 1. A schematic representation of human postural control in quiet stance. To maintain upright position and stabilize the body, there are continuously changing visual, vestibular, proprioceptive and mechanoreceptive sensory inputs. As the standing human is an unstable physical structure there can be stable static position. Stance is therefore maintained by dinamic feedback control with contribution of anticipatory or feed forward, information

Posturography Without Perturbations

Measurement of body movements to quantitatively and objectively evaluate postural control and responses led to the development of different sets of posturography. The basic concept depends on measurement of the forces actuated by the feet against the ground, measured with a forceplate. The forceplate consists of force transducers placed to pick up the distribution of forces which are vertical or horizontal to the ground. The simultaneous recordings from several transducers allows calculation of the moment produced by the standing human in different directions and shear (or transitional) forces to normalize effects of weight of different subjects. The data may then be used to calculate the projection of forces against the ground. It is of utmost importance to the understanding of posturography to realize that the recorded projection of all forces against the ground are not the same as a projection of the subject centre of mass (or gravity) but just the centre of forces. The trace that is recorded is thus not equivalent to movements, especially fast ones, but rather to the stabilizing forces.

Different variables may be derived from the force measurements. The sway amplitude, sway variance, of sway in either anteroposterior or lateral planes or sway path, sway velocity, sway area describing two-dimensional movements are commonly used variables to evaluate postural competence [2]. Although measurements of quiet stance may contribute to separation of groups of subjects with different lesions, the normal variations are so wide that classification of individual responses and, hence, clinical usefulness, becomes ambiguous. To master such shortcomings, different techniques to increase the demands on the postural control are applied [2]. The idea is that if there is a deficit in the postural control system that is not evident because of the redundancy and adaptability of the systems, the deficit will become evident if further sensory information is lost or distorted. The classical Romberg test uses evasion of visual clues to load the postural system. Likewise, posturography can be performed and results compared with open and closed eyes. This is a standard procedure used in most test set-ups (for review see [2, 3, 14]). If the increase of sway compared to normals is greater with open eyes than with closed eyes, this might be taken as suggesting less effective use of visual clues and may be, but not unequivocally, interpreted as a sign of decreased CNS function. A foam rubber pad can be positioned between the feet of the subject and the forceplate to reduce mechanoreceptor sensation from the soles of the feet and increase the difficulties in stabilizing the body [14-16]. The patient can be asked to place his head in different positions to increase difficulties with vestibular cervical interaction [14, 17].

The sensory integration tests of the Equitest equipment, which is probably the most widespread commercially available equipment, utilize six sets of disturbed sensory information to estimate a sensory integration set [18]. In conditions one, two and three the subjects stand on a stable platform and the anteroposterior sway is estimated in percentage of maximal sway. In condition one the subjects stand with open eyes, in condition two with closed eyes; in condition three the visual surroundings move with the moving centre of pressure executed by the feet to distort the visual information on the movement. In conditions four to six the platform reacts on the pressure applied on it, i.e. when the forces actuated by the feet move forwards, the platform rotates in a toes-down direction. In condition four the subjects stand with open eyes, in condition five with closed eyes; in condition six the visual surrounding move with the moving centre of pressure executed by the feet to distort the visual information on the movement (compare with conditions one to three above). Conditions five and six are the most difficult to endure and decreased results in those are said to constitute a vestibular pattern. Deficits in conditions three, five and six are considered a sensory integration deficit and may be expected in some posterior fossa lesions. There have not yet been reports to the authors knowledge of correlation between specific patterns and posterior fossa lesions.

Posturography with Induced Perturbations

To further load human postural control with the purpose of revealing deficits, the standing subject may be exposed to different perturbations and the responses to recover quiet stance are evaluated. In the T-Post system from Toennies the subjects stand, leaning somewhat backwards, the platform then tilts and induces a further backward movement of the body. The subjects have to move forward to avoid falling; latencies, and amplitudes of this movement can be combined with EMG recordings to estimate response latencies. The method can detect movement and probe synergistic muscle activity if combined with EMG. In the motor coordination test of the Equitest the platform is either tilted or translated with different velocities and the postural reactions of the subject are measured. The diagnostic power of this procedure in posterior fossa lesions has not yet been reported to the knowledge of the author. Vibration toward the antigravity muscles induces a sensation of movement and involuntary body movements [19]. This has been used to perturb the standing human for diagnostic purposes, calculating vibration induced body sway (VBS) [20]. Patients with posterior fossa lesions are reported to have larger responses when vibrated toward neck muscles than calf muscles, compared to subjects with vestibular lesions. Vibration toward the calf muscles according to a pseudorandom binary stimulus (PRBS) induces an on-and off-going perturbation which can be used to estimate an input-output relation and model postural control, which allows estimation of so-called characteristic parameters of postural control [21]. Comparing these parameters one can get an estimation of the postural control of the subject. Recently, it has been suggested that the use of these parameters can distinguish, for example, between an acoustic neurinoma and an acute vestibular lesion and also distinguish subjects with cervical disorders. Patients who recover from hemispheric stroke demonstrate remaining differences in postural control when evaluated with those parameters [4]. A vestibular spinal perturbation may evoke both lateral and anteroposterior body sway [16] by galvanic stimulation of the vestibular nerves. Evaluation of these responses may give further information in posterior fossa lesions but so far clinical studies are lacking. Visual stimulation inducing a sensation of small amplitude translatory movements of the surroundings may induce perturbations in the anteroposterior plane, which, not surprisingly, differs in subjects with cerebellar lesions [22]. The effect of visual stimulation, however, may be dependent on attention and state of mind and different patterns of response may be assumed in normal subjects. So far visually induced perturbations, with the exception of the so-called stabilized visual frame in Equitest measurements, have not been used in clinical routine to the knowledge of the author.

Discussion

At present, assessment of postural function seems to be becoming increasingly important for the evaluation of the patient with a suspected posterior fossa lesion as well as other patients with suspected disturbed postural function. Although most tests are dependent on cooperation of the patient and the fact that a pathologic outcome may not contribute a clear-cut anatomical location of a suspected lesion, the tests give information about the functional deficits induced by a lesion. In combination with objective assessment of vestibular and eye motor function, measurements of postural control may, however, strengthen or reduce suspicions of posterior fossa lesions. It should again be emphasized that such tests evaluate the functional effect of lesions while neuroimaging may contribute further information on the specific anatomical localization. Knowledge of the extent of such functional deficit is of importance for the overall approach to the patient's disorder. Furthermore, evaluation of postural control before, during and after therapy contributes information about the effect of treatment or rehabilitation. There are several automatic and computerized approaches available and ongoing development and refinement of methods. It is, however, the author's opinion that if such methods are not available, the use of functional scales and careful clinical examinations should not be disregarded.

References

1. Johansson R, Magnusson M, Åkesson M (1988) Identification of human posture dynamics IEEE. Trans Biomed Eng 35:858-869
2. Johansson R, Magnusson M (1991) Human postural dynamics. CRC Crit Rev Biomed Eng 18:413-437
3. Dietz V (1992) Human neuronal control of automatic functional movements: interaction between central programs and afferent input. Physiol Rev 72 1:33-69
4. Magnusson M, Johansson K, Johansson BB (1994) Sensory stimulation promotes normalization of postural control after stroke. Stroke 25:1176-1180
5. Silfverskiöld BP (1977) Cortical cerebellar degeneration associated with a specific disorder of standing and locomotion. Acta Neurol Scand 55:257
6. Lindmark B, Hamrin E (1988) Evaluation of functional capacity after stroke as a basis for active intervention. Scand J Rehab Med 20:103-109

7. Gabell A, Simmons MB (1982) Balance coding. Phys Ther 68:286-288
8. Tinetti ME (1986) Performance-oriented assessment of mobility problems in elderly patients. J Am Geriatr Soc 34:119-126
9. Horak FB (1987) Clinical measurement of postural control in adults. Phys Ther 67:1881-1885
10. Berg KO, Maki BE, Williams JI, Holliday PJ, Wood-Dauphinee SL (1992) Clinical and laboratory measures of postural balance in an elderly population. Arch Phys Med Rehabil 73:1073-1080
11. Duncan PW, Weiner DK, Chandler J, Studenski S (1990) Functional reach: a new clinical measure of balance. J Gerontol 45:192-197
12. Ekdahl C, Jarnlo GB, Andersson SI (1989) Standing balance in healthy subjects. Evaluation of a quantitative test battery on a force platform. Scand J Rehabil Med 21:187-195
13. Östlund H (1979) A study of aim and strategy of stability control in quasistationary standing. Thesis, Deptartment of Neurology and Research, St. Lars Sjukhus, Lund
14. Norré ME (1990) Posture in otoneurology, vol 1. Acta Otorhinolaryngol (Belg) 44:55-181
15. Brandt T (1988) Sensory function and posture. Posture and gait. Exerpta medica. International congress series 812:127-136
16. Magnusson M, Enbom H, Johansson R, Wiklund J (1991) Significance of pressor input from the feet in lateral postural control - the effect of hypothermia on galvanically induced body sway. Acta Otolaryngol (Stockh) 110:321-327
17. Lund S, Broberg C (1983) Effects of different head positions on postural sway in man induced by a reproducible vestibular error signal. Acta Physiol Scand 117 (2):307-309
18. Horak FB, Nashner LM (1986) Central programming of postural movements: adaptation to altered support-surface configurations. J Neurophysiol 55 (6):1369-1381
19. Eklundh G (1971) Some physical properties of muscle vibrators used to elicit tonic proprioceptive reflexes in man. Acta Soc Med Upsal 76:271-279
20. Aalto H, Pyykkö I, Starck J (1988) Computerized posturography, a development of the measuring system. Acta Otolaryngol Suppl (Stockh) 449:71-75
21. Pyykkö I, Enbom H, Magnusson M, Schalén L (1991) Effect of proprioceptor stimulation on postural stability in patients with peripheral or central vestibular lesion. Acta Otolaryngol (Stockh) 111 (1):27-35
22. Bronstein AM, Hood JD, Gresty MA, Panagi C, (1990) Visual control of balance in cerebellar and parkinsonian syndromes. Brain 113:767-779

Posturography and Vertigo

P. L. Ghilardi, A. Casani and B. Fattori

Traumatic damage to the soft tissue in the neck may cause the onset of vertigo and dizziness in a large number of cases [13, 31, 47, 49]. The attacks of vertigo and dizziness may last for months after the injury, although these usually decrease significantly as the neck pain subsides. The dizzy symptoms which follow even a rather light case of whiplash injury (WI) are usually described in non-specific terms such as lightheadedness, off-balance, and floating and only a small percentage of patients have a sensation of spinning or rotatory vertigo [1].

In the majority of the cases, WI may be accompanied by a number of subjective symptoms (neck pain, headache, shoulder pain, visual disturbancies, tinnitus, lack of energy, unsteadiness, lightheadedness, and so on), but the objective signs are often very poor [31].

WI can be considered as a trauma affecting the tissue around the cervical vertebrae and not as a lesion of the bone. The damage causes a strain or sprain in the muscles, ligaments, fascias, tendons, etc., but the reaction of these tissues involved (hemorrages, edema, etc.) develops rather slowly. This is the reason why patients suffering from WI start complaining of their symptoms (particularly dizziness and vertigo) some time after the accident.

The explanation of the vertiginous symptoms resulting from WI is based on various hypothetical pathogeneses such as compression of the proximal vertebral artery against the transverse process of the seventh cervical vertebra [13, 30], a proprioceptive mechanism [3, 14] or a sympathetic origin [27]. This latter hypothesis is based on the assumption of an overexcitation of the cervical and lumber proprioceptors.

WI can affect the balance system throughby an involvement of one or more of these structures: (1) the neck proprioceptors; (2) the peripheral vestibular system; (3) the central vestibular system.

After WI, an abrupt increase in discharge from the neck proprioceptors, usually asymmetric, might be generated by an overexcitation of the sympathetic fibres related to the ß receptors of the deep cervical erector muscles

Institute of Otorhinolaryngology, University of Pisa, 56100 Pisa, Italy, Tel. (39)-50-592625, Fax (39)-50-550307

[27, 28]. On the other hand, electrophysiological studies suggest the presence of a cervico-ocular reflex (COR) mediated via the vestibular nuclei [29, 43], where secondary vestibular neurons show a convergence of neck and semicircular canal afferents, demostrating a strict interaction between COR and vestibulo-ocular reflex (VOR). The above-mentioned anatomo-functional connections between the cervical afferents and the vestibular system might explain the onset of vertigo after WI, resulting from an abnormal centripetal input from the cervical muscles which not only can affect the vestibular nuclei and, eventually, the cerebellum, but can also, via the reticulo-spinal tract, produce some effects on the spinal cord causing ataxia and postural instability.

The peripheral vestibular system might be damaged after a WI due to mechanical effects (such as labyrinthine commotion) causing both a shaking of the inner ear induced by the sudden acceleration and also vascular lesions produced by the traumatic effects on the vertebral artery with a subsequent reduction in blood supply to the labyrinth. The otoliths are obviously more vulnerable to sudden accelerations and WI might cause otolith vertigo with or without cupulolithiasis. The disease usually shows a benign course, similar to that of neck pain. The WI might dislodge otoconia from the gelatinous matrix, resulting in different loads on the macula; in this case, the patient describes a non-rotatory vertigo, particularly associated with head extension and an unsteadiness in gait similar to walking on pillows [6].

Furthermore, WI frequently damages the brain: lesions in the nerve fibres and chromatolysis were observed in neurons of the lateral vestibular nucleus, the medullary portion of the reticular formation and even in the red nucleus [16]. These lesions might be due not only to a vascular-mediated damage, but also to a stretching of the neural structures of the cervical spinal cord and the brainstem. On these grounds, vertiginous symptoms after WI will not only be due to labyrinthine or cervical lesions alone but in addition may be frequently caused by brainstem disorders [40, 44, 49].

Regarding the evidence of VOR abnormalities after WI, the literature describes results confirming the relatively high percentage of vestibular and/or oculomotor pathological findings [11, 13, 28, 39, 43, 44, 49]. The positional nystagmus is considered to be the most frequent sign, especially when it appears if the head is turned towards the side injured by WI [44, 45]. There may be also a spontaneous nystagmus and some patients might show a canal paresis on the same side as the WI. Pfaltz [40] states that spontaneous nystagmus is rather uncommon. However, some reports [13, 39, 49] indicate a high incidence of spontanous nystagmus with an amplitude of more than 5°/s in 63% of patients suffering from WI [39]. We must consider these results with caution because spontaneous or positional nystagmus can be found in a high percentage of normal subjects examined with their eyes closed [1].

Positional nystagmus of paroxysmal benign type can be considered a relatively common finding [6, 11, 40] and a persistent positional nystagmus (direction changing) of central type is looked upon as a possible sign of WI in which brainstem involvement might occur [40].

Also an impairment in the eye tracking test is considered a reliable objective sign of vestibular damage after WI [49].

Our previously published reports [11] regarding the results of VOR examination in a group of patients suffering from vertigo as a consequence of WI showed a high percentage (39.9%) of pathological findings (Fig. 1). The damage was considered of peripheral type in 26.4% of the patients and of central type in 12% of all cases. Cervical nystagmus, evoked by the neck torsion test [25], was the most common sign and it was found in 22 (21.5%) of the 102 patients. This result was significantly different from that in the control group of normal subjects ($p > 0.05$). Paroxysmal positional vertigo (PPV) was evident in seven cases (6.8%). No correlation was found between cervical nystagmus and positional stationary nystagmus ($p < 0.001$).This latter nystagmus was found in three patients (3%).

These observations confirm that the "cervical or neck torsion" nystagmus is one of the most interesting topics when the problem of vertigo from WI is discussed.

Conflicting opinions arise regarding the significance of this nystagmus. Despite the fact that many Authors find a nystagmus induced by passive head rotation as a very frequent sign of vestibular involvement of WI [2, 32, 39, 46], there is no convincing evidence that this sign could clearly differen-

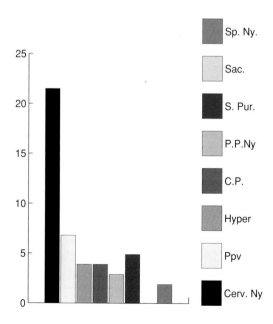

Fig. 1. Percentage of cervico-ocular reflex (COR) and vestibulo-ocular reflex (VOR) abnormalities in 102 patients suffering from vertigo after WI. *Cerv. Ny*: cervical nystagmus; *Ppv*: paroxysmal positional vertigo; *Hyper*: caloric hyperreflexia; *C.P.*: canal paresis; *P.P. Ny*: positional persistent nystagmus; *S. Pur.*: smooth pursuit; *Sac.*: saccades; *Sp. Ny*: spontaneous nystamus of central type

tiate between normal and pathologic subjects [36]. Nevertheless, cervical nystagmus appears as one of the most interesting signs from a theoretical point of view. The search for cervical nystagmus could be a possibility for objective proof of the post-traumatic complaints, especially in younger patients [2]. There is no evidence as yet for this hypothesis. We found cervical nystagmus in about 20% of the patients suffering from vertigo after WI [11], but other Authors [2, 39] have reported higher incidences. Therefore, this nystagmus may be one of the most significant signs for the evaluation of post-traumatic vertigo.

It has also been suggested that patients suffering from the worst conditions of postural instability are those who show a clear neck torsion nystagmus [21]. This observation further complicates the theoretical speculations regarding vertigo, posture and WI. No correlation seems to exist between the extent of the traumatic damage in the neck and the presence of cervical nystagmus. As a matter of fact, the evidence for cervical nystagmus has to hold other factors in due consideration, whether pre-existing or subsequent to WI, such as labyrinthine function. We can conclude that at present we do not exactly know which and how various mechanisms work in the genesis of cervical nystagmus.

On the basis of previous reports, we can postulate that vertigo is a commom symptom after WI, but a retrospective analysis of abnormal oculomotor findings such as spontaneous, positional or cervical nystamus shows little or uncertain clinical significance [1].

Post-traumatic vertigo is not a clinical entity, but this term refers only to the common etiology of a heterogeneous collection of vestibular disorders [6]. Even if there are many convincing signs indicating the existence of anatomical and functional connections between the neck and the vestibular system, the assessment of vertigo after WI is extremely complex. No reliable clinical, electronystagmographic or posturographic test exists to confirm the linkage between the neck trauma and the vertiginous symptoms. However, the incidence of vertigo and dizziness after WI is surprisingly high [11, 28, 30, 31, 36, 39, 40, 44, 49] and an otoneurologic study is strongly recommended.

As already emphasised, several structures and functions are involved in WI; in most cases we can reveal a combined mixture of central, peripheral and cervical lesions. Hence, an atypical vertigo, not rotatory, even an aspecific sensation of dizziness, is the most common complaint which occurs in the majority of cases. Furthermore when the VOR imbalance signs disappear, the postural instability is usually still present in a large number of patients and it lasts for a long time as a consequence of the vestibulo-spinal reflex (VSR) disorder.

Keeping these observations in mind, static posturography could provide useful information about the postural conditions of patients suffering from vertigo after WI.

Keeping erect standing position is a very complicated process which aims at achieving a stable relationship between one's own body and the surrounding environment. It entails neural mechanisms which coordinate both the posture of the individual body segments and the equilibrium on the whole. A perfect balance is obtained when the center of gravity, better defined as the projection of the mass center, is at the center of the body. Posture is due to the activity of motoneurons and encephalic centers but also to sensory information coming from peripheral receptors which are integrated by brainstem centers (mainly at reticular and cerebellar area levels). Balance function is obtained through the elaboration of sensory inputs provided by visual and vestibular systems and by proprioception (especially from the cervico-facial tract and lower limb muscles and articulations) [41].

Up until now, an otoneurologic examination was mainly performed with the evaluation of the VOR through specific and well-codified techniques. Equilibrium is now considered more often, since it is evident that the VSR plays a fundamental role in the maintenance of an upright standing position. VOR has the task of stabilizing the visual field. VSR is the nervous reflex that helps muscles to counterbalance gravity. Postural function is maintnance of the erect standing position which is dynamically threatened by gravity and by both voluntary and involuntary movement of the head and body. Moreover, posture stabilizes the visual field by balancing the head. In order to achieve these goals, compensating movements are automatically elaborated by the reflex arcs controlled by the brainstem centers and the cerebellum receiving proprioceptive, visual and vestibular information, which communicates the exact position of the body in every moment [38] (Fig. 2). Therefore, a complete study of the

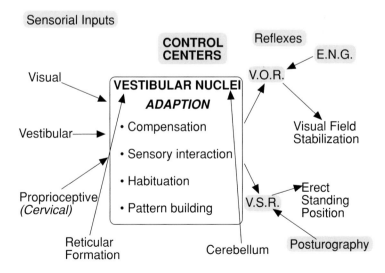

Fig. 2. Scheme of the balance function

124

vestibular and postural functions is not attainable though a routine examination of the VOR, as it cannot provide us with information on the VSR status.

Before the introduction of computerized posturography (PG) [10, 19, 20, 26, 38], the VSR was studied using various tests (Romberg, Fukuda, Unterberger, Babinski-Weil, Ataxia test battery, etc.) which nevertheless do not permit a quantitative and objective study of postural function. Stabilometry has superceded the above mentioned methods by providing objective data which allow a periodical study and comparison of the postural equilibrium in individuals patients and the postural balance in several subjects.

Routinely, PG recording is performed under two basic conditions: (1) patient standing on the platform with eyes open (EO); (2) patient standing on the platform with eyes closed (EC).

Besides these basic tests to verify the presence of a latent postural disorder, other destabilizing tests are usually employed. We use two types of examinations to verify this: (1) patient standing on the platform with EC and with the head in extreme retroflexion (EC-HER) [22]; (2) patient standing on the platform with EC immediately after head shaking (EC-HST) [23].

The parameters we can achieve from the computer elaboration are shown in Table 1.

An important difference between the PG and the older techniques for the study of posture is that the former provides us with precise objective data which can be compared throughout time for each patient and each with different pathologies of balance. Of course, considering the complexity of postural function it might be necessary to carry out other specific tests in order to determine which one of the inputs has the main pathogenic role. For example, by using vibration stimuli on the neck or on lower limb muscles [35], or by reducing the blood flow to the inferior extremities [15], we can evalu-

Table 1. The main parameters and the graphic elaborations obtained by computerized stabilometry

Parameters	Graphic elaborations
X min, max, mean	Displacement of pressure center on X axis
X min, max, mean	Displacement of pressure center on Y axis
Velocity of the sway	Its standard deviation is an index of the "homogeneity" of the postural oscillations
Length L (mm)	Total sway path of center of pressure
Surface S (mm^2)	Is indicative of the precision of the system
L.F.S.	Correlation function between L and S
Statokinesigram	Area covered by the sway
Stabilogram	Displacement on time of the sway for X and Y
Fast Fourier transform	
Romberg's index	Ratio between the same value with EC and EO

ate the role of the proprioceptive inputs in patients suffering from postural disorders. This allows a quantification of the importance of the pressoceptor system for balance and provides us with useful information for the management of rehabilitation treatment.

As already discussed, the cervical area mediates two reflexes by means of the activity of the neck proprioceptors: the COR and the postural neck reflexes whose task is to enable head movement to occur without causing postural imbalance [42, 34]. In humans, neck postural reflexes contribute to posture in strict correlation with other multisensory mechanisms [18], thus making it difficult to carry out a selective and reliable clinical test for the evaluation of the role of the neck in the maintenance of static posture.

In this context, PG, performed with particular types of stimuli or provocation tests, may identify a cervical origin of the dizzy symptoms. Through tests performed with rotation ("cervical dynamic activation") [51], "head turned" [19] (Fig. 3) and retroflexion of the head [7, 14, 21, 37] (Fig. 4), it will be possible to obtain some information on how cervical inputs can generate instability syndromes. However, positive results obtained with the abovementioned tests must be evaluated within the entire clinical context, because they cannot be considered as pathognomonic.

We studied a group of patients suffering from vertigo and dizziness from WI using PG performed in EC and EC-EHR. The results were compared with those obtained in a group of patients suffering from cervical spondylosis and a group of normal subjects. In patients suffering from WI the value of length (L) and surface (S) in EC-HER conditions was abnormal in 87% of the cases, and the Romberg index (RI) (EC-HER/EC) showed a similar result with a significant difference with the other group of patients (Fig. 5). We observed a rather common abnormality in the statokinesigram (SKG) with a marked increase of the S more than the L, indicating poor accuracy of the postural system (Fig. 6) [21]. However, retroflexion of the head might be considered just as effective a manoeuvre to evaluate an irritative condition of the neck proprioceptors; there is also a possibility that the results of the test might be abnormal because of the presence of an otolithic pathology such as the traumatic otolith vertigo [6]. It must to be mentioned that the lesion may not be limited to cervical receptors alone but that it could occasionally also involve the peripheral vestibular system, as well as the central vestibular system (although less frequently). In our experience, unilateral vestibular lesions were recorded in 6% of cases, while bilateral vestibular paresis appeared very rarely [11].

By means of PG we can obtain useful information regarding the postural behaviour of patients suffering from vestibular pathology following a WI.

In the case of *unilateral vestibular lesion* (UVL) immediately after the acute phase, the alterations in the SKG and stabilogram (SBG) are more evident in EO conditions with an increase in the oscillation frequency and a

126

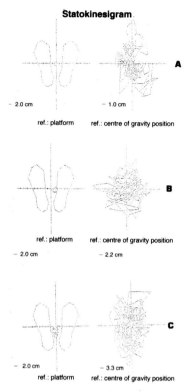

Fig. 3 A-C. Patient suffering from vertigo from WI. **A** Normal result in EO. **B** The SKG is abnormal when the head of the patient is rotated towards the right. **C** A similar pattern can be observed with the head rotated to left

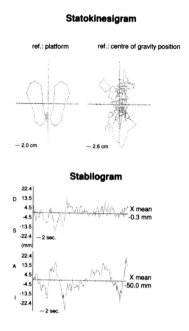

Fig. 4. Patient suffering from WI. *Above*, the pathological SKG in EO-HER; *below*, the SBG shows a prevalence of the oscillation on the anterior-posterior axis

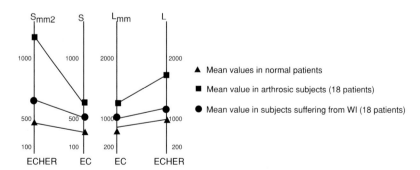

Fig. 5. Increase in the mean values of length (*L*) and surface (*S*) in EC and EC-HER

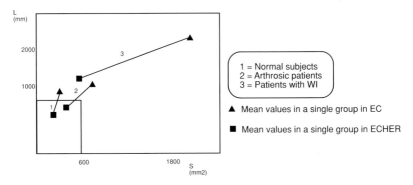

Fig. 6. Comparison between the length *(L)* and the surface *(S)* mean values in EC and EC-HER. The *small square* on the left represents the normal values in EC

displacement of the pressure center towards the affected side and posteriorly (Fig. 7). The fast Fourier transform (FFT) will often show a maximal frequency peak ranging from 0.2 to 0.4 Hz (the resonance frequency of the human pendulum) and this will show a serious deficiency in postural control [48, 52]. As vestibular compensation develops the postural performance improves progressively, even if in certain patients we can notice a backward displacement of the pressure center as if they were suffering from axial extensor muscle rigidity [17]. Often it is only through sensitization tests (EC-HST, EC-HER) that it is possible to detect latent static postural deficiencies not evident in basic conditions (EO and EC) (Fig. 8) [23]. Moreover, the PG allows assessing when some patients have reached a normal postural performance even if there had been previous evidence of incomplete VOR compensation (for example, a positive head shaking test). However, it is also possible to find patients with a high ataxic component of instability even perfectly VOR-compensated [4, 22, 38]. This observation is of primary importance in patients suffering from sequelae of WI. Probably, abnormal proprioceptive input from the neck represents the eliciting stimuli causing alteration in postural stability.

In cases of *bilateral vestibulopathies* following WI, where instability is one of the main symptoms, the PG allows a quantification of the postural deficiency [12]. In this pathology, proprioceptive and visual inputs mainly rule the static posture (Fig. 9). An increase in backward-forward sway with a periodicity of 0.4 Hz can be detected [50]. Frequently, a marked increase in length can be observed only through destabilizing tests [33].

As already mentioned, *PPV* can be considered a relatively common finding after WI. The postural abnormality in patients suffering from PPV has been called "otolithic vertigo". It is caused by different forces acting on the two maculae after the detachment of one part of the otoliths [9]. In 50% of PPV cases, a stabilometric irregularity is recorded with the head in extreme

128

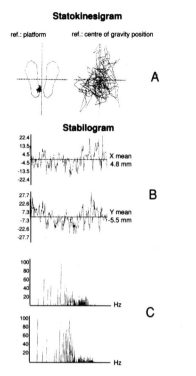

Statokinesigram

ref.: platform   ref.: centre of gravity position

A

Stabilogram

22.4
13.5
4.5
-4.5   X mean
-13.5   4.8 mm
-22.4

B

27.7
22.6
7.3   Y mean
-7.3   -5.5 mm
-22.6
-27.7

100
80
60
40
20
            Hz
                                    C
100
80
60
40
20
            Hz

Statokinesigram

ref.: platform   ref.: centre of gravity position

A

— 2.0 cm   — 4.3 cm

B

— 2.0 cm   — 3.0 cm

C

— 2.0 cm   — 4.3 cm

Fig. 7 A-C. Patient suffering from acute UVL after a WI. **A** The SKG in EO shows a marked increase of S and L with a shift of the centre of pressure towards the left. **B** The SBG shows a marked increase of the oscillation's frequency. **C** The FFT shows a maximal frequency peak on 0.2-0.4 Hz

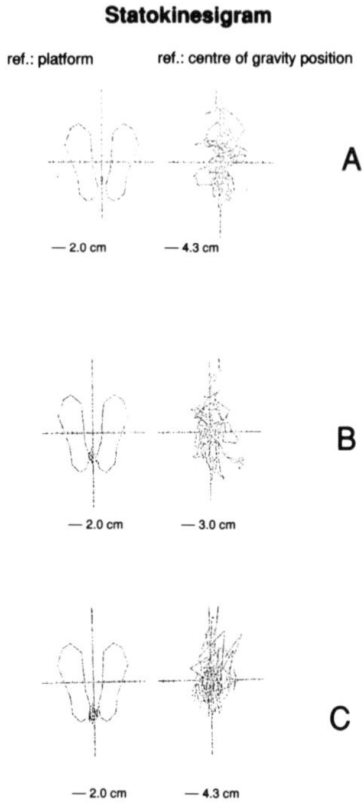

Fig. 8 A-C. Patient suffering from UVL after a WI with EO (**A**) stabilometry is normal. Only with EO-HST (**B**) can an abnormality of SKG be detected. With EO-HER (**C**) postural stability shows a marked worsening

retroflexion. Under these conditions a remarkable increase in the oscillations on the Y axis and a displacement of the pressure center towards the critical side are detected (Fig. 10) [5]. The recovery of PPV through canalith repositioning manoeuvres determines a normalization of the stabilometric performance [5].

In patients suffering from WI in whom *lesions of the central vestibular system* were found, no specific pattern was described regarding their postural behaviour. In most of these cases a serious instability could be recorded: oscillations increased often without well defined laterality with a major increase in S values and often with little variation to the parameters with EO and EC (Fig. 11) [8, 24].

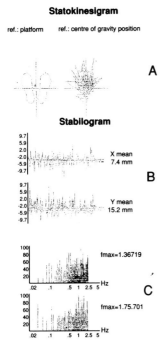

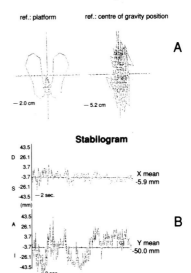

Fig. 9 A-C. Patient suffering from bilateral vestibular paresis after a WI. The SKG with EC (**A**) has a normal S but an anterior shift of the centre of pressure is detectable together with an increase of L. The SBG (**B**) shows a very marked increase of the oscillation and the FFT (**C**) has a maximal frequency peak of 1.3-1.7

Fig. 10 A, B. Patient suffering from PPV after WI. The SKG with OC-HER (**A**) is abnormal; the SBG (**B**) shows a prevalence of the oscillation on the anterior-posterior axis

Nevertheless, it must be considered that the findings may be altered or modified because of the combined actions of more than one degree of lesion.

Beside a definition of the postural damage, static PG allows visualizing and quantifying the extent of the disease and the effects of therapy on postural behavior in patients with VSR deficiency.

This observation has to be kept in mind in the case of patients suffering from postural abnormalities following WI in whom the posturographic test performed in EC-HER plays an important role for evaluating the significance of the cervical proprioceptive input at the base of the vertiginous symptoms.

In this framework, PG seems to be very useful for monitoring both postural deficiencies and the subsequent therapy.

130

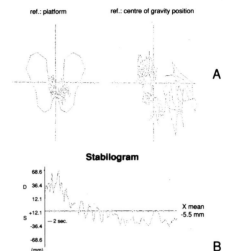

Fig. 11 A, B. Patient suffering from a lesion of the central vestibular system following WI. The SKG (A) shows a pathological increase of surface more than length. The SBG (B) shows a shift towards the left side

References

1. Baloh RW, Honrubia V (1990) Clinical neurophysiology of the vestibular system. 2nd ed, FA Davis Company, Philadelphia
2. Becker R, Meyer E (1991) Cervical syndrome due to trauma. In: Claussen CF, Kirtane MV (eds). Vertigo, nausea, tinnutus and hypoacusia due to head and neck trauma. Elsevier Science Publ, Amsterdam, pp 259-263
3. Biemond A, De Jong JMBV (1969) On cervical nystagmus and related disorders. Brain 92:437-458
4. Bles W, DeJong JMBV (1986) Uni- and bilateral loss of vestibular function. In: Bles W, Brandt T (eds). Disorders of posture and gait. Elsevier, Amsterdam, pp 127-140
5. Boniver R (1991) Posturographie et vertige paroxystique bénin. Acta ORL Belg 45:331-334
6. Brandt T (1991) Vertigo. Its multisensory syndromes. Springer-Verlag, London
7. Brandt T, Krapczyk S, Malbenden L (1981) Postural imbalance with head extension. Improvement by training as a model for ataxia therapy. Ann NY Acad Sc 374:646-649
8. Brandt T, Dieterich M, Buchele W (1986) Postural abnormalities in central vestibular brain stem lesions. In: Bles W, Brandt T (eds). Disorders of posture and

gait. Elsevier, Amsterdam, pp 141-156

9. Buchele W, Brandt T (1986) Benign paroxysmal positioning vertigo and posture. In: Bles W, Brandt T (eds). Disorders of posture and gait. Elsevier, Amsterdam, pp 101-112

10. Casani A, Ghilardi PL, Pardini L, Fattori B, Piragine F (1989) La piattaforma stabilometrica: sua utilità nella strategia diagnostica otoneurologica. In: Ghilardi PL, Piragine F (eds). Analisi computerizzata della reazione suolo-piede nelle alterazioni dell'equilibrio posturale e della deambulazione: approccio interdisciplinare. TEP Edizioni, Pisa, pp 19-27

11. Casani A, Ghilardi PL, Fattori B, Vannucchi R (1991) The neuro-otological findings following mild head injury. In: Claussen CF, Kirtane MV (eds). Vertigo, nausea, tinnutus and hypoacusia due to head and neck trauma. Elsevier Science Publ, Amsterdam, pp 133-136

12. Casani A, Ghilardi PL, Fattori B, Pardini L, Raffi G, Piragine F (1992) Assessment of vestibular and postural testing in patients with bilateral vestibular paresis. In: Motta G (ed). The new frontiers of otorhinolaryngology in Europe. Monduzzi ed, Bologna, pp 369-363

13. Compere WE (1968) Electronystagmographic findings in patients with "whiplash" injury. Laryngoscope 78:1226-1233

14. De Jong JMBV, Bles W (1986) Cervical dizziness and ataxia. In: Bles W, Brandt T (eds). Disorders of posture and gait. Elsevier, Amsterdam, pp 185-206

15. Diener HC, Dichgans J, Guschlbauer B, Mau H (1984) The significance of proprioception on postural stabilization assessed by ischemia. Brain Res 296:103-109

16. Elliot FE (1964) Clinical neurology. WB Saunders, Philadelphia

17. Franchignoni FP, Castelnuovo P, Mevio E, Vanni C, Liverani F (1985) Etude électronystagmographique et posturographique de la névrite vestibulaire. In: Hausler R (ed). Les vertiges d'origine périphérique et centrale. Ipsen Publ, Paris, pp 175-177

18. Fukuda T (1961) Studies on human dynamic postures from the viewpoint of postural reflexes. Acta Otolaryngol [Suppl 161]:1-52

19. Gagey PM, Baron JB, Ushio N (1980) Introduction à la posturologie clinique. Aggressologie 21:119-123

20. Gagey PM (1986) Huit leçons de posturologie. Association Française de Posturologie, Paris

21. Ghilardi PL, Casani A (1989) Approccio posturografico alla vertigine di origine cervicale. Atti LXXVI Congresso Naz SIO, Rieti 24-27 maggio, pp 383-387

22. Ghilardi PL, Fattori B, Casani A, Piragine F (1990) La posturografia nei deficit unilaterali vestibolari periferici. Acta Otorhinol Ital 10:347-346

23. Ghilardi PL, Fattori B, Casani A, Vatteroni UR, Capetta M (1991) L'utilizzo del Head Shaking Test nella diagnostica posturografica. Acta Otorhinol Ital 11:571-577

24. Ghilardi PL, Fattori B, Casani A (1994) Vascular and neoplastic pathologies of the posterior cranial fossa: the role of otoneurology in clinical diagnosis. In: Cesarani A, Alpini D (eds). Equilibrium disorders. Brainstem and cerebellar pathology. Springer-Verlag, Milano, Berlin, pp 106-124

25. Greiner GF, Conraux C, Collard M (1971) Le nystagmus d'origine cervical.

Mise en evidence et interet clinique. Ann Otolaryngol 88:151-167
26. Guidetti G (1989) Stabilometria clinica. Amplifon Edizioni, Milano
27. Hinoki M, Niki H (1975) Neurotological studies on the role of the sympathetic nervous system in the formation of traumatic of vertigo of cervical origin. Acta Otolaryngol [Suppl 330]:185-196
28. Hinoki M (1985) Vertigo due to whiplash injury: a neurotological approach. Acta Otolaryngol [Suppl 419]:9-29
29. Hirosaka O, Maeda M (1972) Cervical effects on abducens motoneurons and their interactions with vestibulo-ocular reflex. Exp Brain Res 18:512-530
30. Jongkees LBW (1969) Cervical vertigo. Laryngoscope 79:1473-1484
31. Jongkees LBW (1983) Whiplash examination. Laryngoscope 93:113-114
32. Hülse M (1983) Die zervicalen gleichgewichtsstörungen. Springer, Berlin
33. Kaga H, Maeda H, Marsh RR (1983) The effect of optical reversal on standing posture to be used as a screening test. Agressologie 24(2):777-778
34. Mergner T, Anastasopoulos D, Becker W (1982) Neuronal responses to horizontal neck deflection in the group X region of the cat's medullary brainstem. Exp Brain Res 45:146-206
35. Nakagawa H, Ohashi N, Watanabe Y, Mizukoshi K (1993) The contribution of proprioception in posture control in normal subjects. Acta Otolaryngol [Suppl 504]:112-116
36. Norré ME, Stevens A (1987) Cervical vertigo. Diagnostic and semiological problems with special emphasis upon "cervical nystmus". Acta ORL Belg 41:436-452
37. Norré ME, Forrez G, Stevens A, Beckers A (1987) Cervical vertigo diagnosed by posturography? Preliminar report. Acta ORL Belg 41:574-582
38. Norré ME (1990) Posture in otoneurology. Acta ORL Belg 44:183-363
39. Oosterveld WJ, Kortschot HW, Kingma GG, de Jong HAA, Saatci MR (1991) Electronystagmographic findings following cervical whiplash injuries. Acta Otolayngol 111:201-205
40. Pfaltz CR (1984) Vertigo in the disorders of the neck. In: Dix MR, Hood JD (eds). Vertigo. John Wiley and Sons, Chicester
41. Roberts TDM (1967) Neurophysiology of postural mechanism. 1st ed, Butterwoths, London
42. Roberts TDM (1973) Reflex balance. Nature 244:158-185
43. Rubin AM, Young JH, Milne AC (1975) Vestibular-neck integration in vestibular nuclei. Brain Res 96:99-102
44. Rubin W (1973) Whiplash with vestibular involvement. Arch Otolaryngol 97:85-87
45. Rubin W (1993) Differential diagnosis of disorders causing dizziness. Am J Otol 14:309-312
46. Scherer H (1985) Halsdebingter schwindel. Arch Oto Rhino Laryngol [Suppl II]:107-124
47. Sturzenegger M, DiStefano G, Radanov B, Schnidrig A (1994) Presenting symptoms and signs after whiplash injury: the influence of accident mechanisms. Neurology 44:688-693
48. Taguki K (1978) Spectral analysis of the movement of the center of gravity in vertiginous and ataxic patients. Agressologie 19B:69-70

49. Toglia JU (1976) Acute flexion-extension injury of the neck: electro-nystagmographic study of 309 patients. Neurology 26:808-814
50. Tokita T, Maeda M, Miyata H (1981) The role of the labyrinth in standing posture regulation. Acta Otolaryngol 91:521-527
51. Vicini C, Rasi F, Valzania F, Neri W (1987) Alterazioni stabilometriche a seguito di attivazione cervicale statica e dinamica. Valori normativi e risultati preliminari nelle patologie del rachide cervicale. In: Di Marco A and Rumiano C (eds). Alterazioni del controllo posturale in età evolutiva e patologie del rachide. Ed Scient Cuzzolin, Avellino
52. Yoneda S, Tokumasu K (1986) Frequency analysis of body sway in the upright posture. Acta Otolaryngol 102:87-92

Diagnosis and Treatment of Equilibrium Disorders in Whiplash Injuries: Posture and Stance Disorders

S. Barozzi and B. Monti

Biomechanics of Standing

The definition of "postural stability" is complex because different components of the equilibrium system are involved (sensory-motor and central nervous system components). In biomechanics a posture is defined as stable when the body's center of gravity (COG) is positioned vertically over the base of support.

For man the "stance" is inevitably unstable because the body COG is located a significant distance (at the height of the lower part of trunk) above a relatively small base of support. Thus, a normal subject with feet in place sways like an upside down pendulum inside the limits of stability. When the COG is positioned above the center of the base of support postural sways may reach the limits of stability without the subject losing his balance.

By contrast, when the COG is offset forward, backward or to one side of the center of support (posture in flexion or in extension as happens in whiplash injuries) the subject is more unstable because he can oscillate less in the direction of the offset without losing balance.

Different stable postures are possible according to the relative position of the three principal muscle-joint systems - ankles, knees and hips - between the body COG and the base of support (Fig. 1).

When external perturbations happen the COG oscillates differently according to the postural movement strategy adopted by each individual, depending on the amplitude of the body's displacement and on individual structural patterns.

The *ankle strategy* is most effective for small COG movemtents: the body acts like a rigid mass and rotates about the ankle joints. This is possible by contracting the ankle, thigh and lower trunk muscles.

The *hip strategy*, in contrast, is mostly used for large COG movements: the body sways moving hips forward and backward with little ankle move-

Servizio Diagnosi e Terapia Turbe dell'Equilibrio, Istituto di Audiologia, Università di Milano, Via Pace, 9, Milan, Italy, Tel. (39)-2-55035218

ment. This generates horizontal reaction forces against the support surface opposite to the direction of hip movement.

The *stepping strategy* operates in order to avoid a fall when the destabilizing force shifts the COG beyond the limits of stability (Fig. 2).

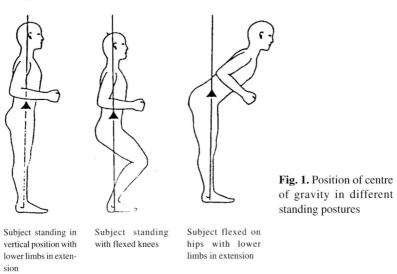

Fig. 1. Position of centre of gravity in different standing postures

Subject standing in vertical position with lower limbs in extension

Subject standing with flexed knees

Subject flexed on hips with lower limbs in extension

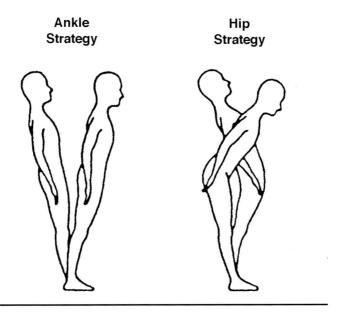

Ankle Strategy

Hip Strategy

Fig. 2. Different strategies to counteract displacements of COG

Equitest: Description of the System

The Equitest system (NeuroCom International, Inc; Clockamas, Oregon) is a dynamic posturography device which allows different movements of the support surface and different conditions of integration of sensory inputs (Fig. 3). The Equitest system consists of:

- A platform provided with pressure-sensitive strain gauges located in each quadrant. It can translate horizontally forward or backward and rotate about an axis colinear with the ankle joint.
- A movable visual surface which encloses the patient's visual surrounding and rotates about an axis colinear with the ankle joint.
- Computer, monitor and printer which analyze, visualize and print data.

The Equitest standard protocol consists of two tests: (1) the sensory organization test (SOT); (2) the motor control test (MCT).

Sensory Organization Test

The SOT assesses the ability of a subject to use visual, vestibular or somatosensory information to maintain upright stance under different sensory conditions. Tests conditions are meant to isolate the function of each equilibrium sub-system by reducing the contribution of others or by presenting conflicting sensory inputs. Thus, during the test, the platform and the visual surrounding are fixed or rotated proportionally to any forward or backward sway of the subject (sway-referenced support and sway-referenced visual surrounding) according to the following six combinations (Fig. 4):

1. Normal vision   (fixed support)
2. Absent vision   (fixed support)
3. Sway-referenced vision   (fixed support)
4. Normal vision   (sway-referenced support)
5. Absent vision   (sway-referenced support)
6. Sway-referenced vision   (sway-referenced support)

Information from a sense subjected to *sway-referencing* suggests that the orientation of the body COG relative to gravity is not changing when in fact it is. Normally, individuals ignore a sway-referenced sensory input and maintain balance by using other sensory inputs.

In addition to sway-referencing, *eyes-closed* conditions are used to further isolate the somatosensory and vestibular systems. The original test scheme doesn't reduce or confound the contribution of the vestibular system. *Head extension* may also be useful because it places the utricular otolith organs in a disadvantageous position. Several Authors have stressed head extension as a method to reduce the utricular otolith component. Besides

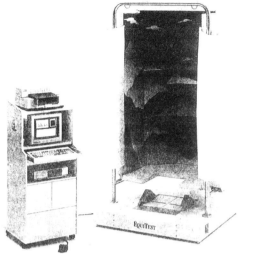

Fig. 3. The Equitest system

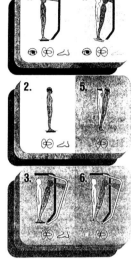

Fig. 4. Ther sensory organization test

causing unfavorable placement of the utricular otoliths, head extension also enhances cervical proprioceptive input; therefore it could be favourably employed in testing balance of whiplash-injured patients.

A computerized system evaluates COG sways and calcutates, for each test, the *equilibrium score*, comparing the patient's maximum anterior to posterior COG displacement to the theoretical maximum displacement of 12.5°.

The Equitest analysis program also calculates:
- The *composite score*, the avarage of all conditions' scores (Fig. 5).
- *Sensory analysis*, which allows identification of a sensory disfunction and/or an abnormal sensory preference by calculating the ratios of different sensory conditions (Fig. 6).
- The *strategy* of movement adopted to maintain upright stance (ankle strategy - hip strategy) (Fig. 7).
- The *COG alignment* (Fig. 8).

Motor Control Test

The MCT studies automatic postural responses to unexpected movements of the base of support: small, medium and large backward translations; small, medium and large forward translations. Each trial is analyzed in terms of *latency*, *amplitude* and *symmetry* of response. When the support surface is

138

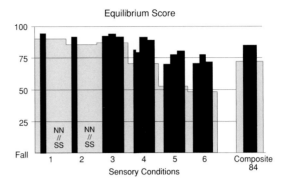

Fig. 5. The composite score

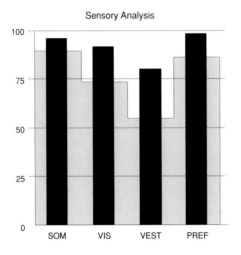

Fig. 6. The sensory analysis

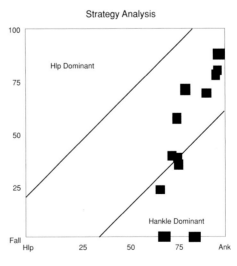

Fig. 7. The strategy analysis (ankle dominant)

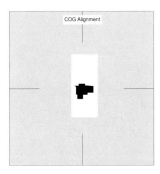

Fig. 8. The COG alignment

unexpectedly translated forward or backward, the body initially remains stationary and becomes offset relative to the base of support. The stiffness of ankle joints initially resists to the sway but is insufficient to stabilize the COG sway.

In *backward* translations, when the *ankle* strategy is used to counteract the forward displacement, a sequential activation of distal to proximal extensor muscles is adopted (gastrocnemius - hamstrings - paraspinal muscles). These muscle activations help to stabilize knee and hip joints so that the body moves as a coordinated unit about the ankle joint.

When the *hip* strategy is used we observe an activation of the flexor muscles of the hip joint (quadriceps and abdominals) that moves the body backward.

In *forward* translations, when the *ankle* strategy is used, we assist with a sequential activation of distal to proximal flexor muscles (tibialis ant., quadriceps and abdominals).

In the *hip* strategy the hip joint moves forward to activat paraspinal muscles and hamstrings.

In the MCT the platform is also tilted abruptly up and down to evaluate adaptation to disruptive balance forces.

Toes up rotations of the support surface stimulate proprioceptors in the gastrocnemius muscles of both legs and elicit muscle forces which tend to destabilize posture. The adaptation test asses the patient's ability to ignore these disruptive somatosensory inputs within five trials (Fig. 9).

Equitest: Use in Whiplash Injuries

The Equitest is a modern device which provides an objective assessment of balance function in its entirety.

With the *composite score* we have an individual global equilibrium measure which can be compared to the average score of clinically normal individuals of the same age.

140

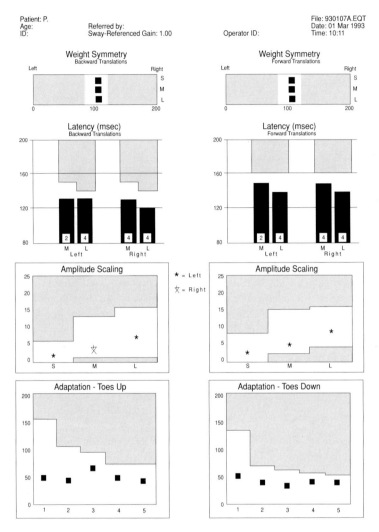

Fig. 9. The motor control test

Several studies made in the normal population confirmed the confidence and the repeatability of computerized dynamic posturography results.

Our experience in evaluating whiplash injuries has showed that in the SOT the composite score can separate, in a confident manner, *normal* subjects at a conventional neurotologic evaluation from *pathological* ones. The only discordance was given by benign positional vertigo results which can be normal at SOT.

The opportunity to have available, objective and repeatable data is important in medical-legal cases following whiplash injuries.

For this purpose computerized dynamic posturography can detect patients who exaggerate symptoms of unsteadiness when test results are physiologically inconsistent. In our experience, in case of deliberate exaggeration of symptoms, we found one or more of the following inconsistent patterns:

1. Composite scores lower than 42% in subjects who don't have ataxia and ambulate without the use of balance aids;
2. Better performances under more difficult conditions (4 - 5 - 6) then under easier ones (1 - 2 - 3).
3. Declining performances during successive trials, with a percentage of equilibrium in the first trial at least two standard deviations greater than the third.
4. Sinusoidal sway traces of COG.
5. Dispersion of the x - y plots of the initial COG alignment.
6. Sudden falls after periods of relative stability in the SOT.
7. Abnormal adaptation in toes-up and toes-down rotation.

In our experience, the 70% of patients with cervical distorstional trauma and with an abnormal composite score and consistent test show vestibular dysfunction patterns on SOT sensory snalysis (the sensory ratio of conditions 5/1 is abnormal).

With somatosensory and visual inputs misleading and unavailable, such as in condition 5, the upright position is allowed by otolith vestibular function which controls the extensor antigravity muscles. Therefore vestibular inputs assessed by sensory analysis are prevalently from the otolith rather than from the canal organs. For this reason in patients with peripheral vestibular disorders Equitest results don't always agree with caloric tests.

So, the abnormal vestibular function found in most patients with cervical trauma can be explained by a deficit in the extensor antigravity muscles.

The motor control *strategy* most commonly observed in sequences of whiplash injuries is the ankle strategy. This is evident in the strategy analysis where points fall along a nearly vertical line on the right of the plot. This finding means that patients are abnormally dependent on ankle movements even when the amplitude of sway approaches the limits of stability.

In patients who underwent whiplash injuries, trauma directed to the cervical spine usually reverberates along the whole column causing a hypofunction of the erector muscles and a prevalence of the flexors which moves forward the body COG.

In order to resist the tendency of falling forward and to move the COG inside the base of support, some corrective postural arrangements are used: forward trunk flexion on the hip with consequent hip stiffness or flexion on the knees.

The choice of a strategy for balancing COG movements depends on personal past experiences, on the individual history of previous accidents and preexistent muscle and joint impairments.

Therefore, although the ankle strategy is the most common pattern in cervical traumas, this doesn't mean that it must be found in all patients with whiplash injuries.

In interpreting Equitest results the strategy analysis can influence the choice of rehabilitative treatment: in cases of prevailing ankle strategy we adopt exercises aimed at potentiating the extensor muscles and only afterwards exercises with the purpose of recovering hip mobility.

In MCT the evaluation of *latency* offers interesting considerations: latencies within normal ranges are observed either in forward or in backward translations only in a limited number of patients with whiplash injuries. In our experience 86% of patients have abnormal latencies either in forward (10%) or in backward translations (12%) or in both (64%). Response strength scores and weight symmetry have always been normal. In whiplash injuries abnormal latencies can be explained as disorders in the afferent somatosensory pathways.

Medico-legal Aspects

R. BONIVER

Introduction

The legal redress for bodily injury goes back to the very ancient concept of "Eye for an eye - tooth for a tooth". It is really a kind of revenge fee for body lesions. The financial compensation is the civilised way to restore justice.

The need for a referee to avoid excess compensation has quickly appeared. This referee is the expert. He has to be neutral and must detail the extent of the lesions.

When it comes to evaluating bodily injury, not only are the same terms concerning invalidity, incapacity, etc., not used throughout the various countries, but also the same terms - for example, invalidity, have a different sense from one country to the other. The laws and their interpretations are also different.

According to these arguments, it is not our purpose to define a disability scale, but we do think that a common approach to the medico-legal problem is necessary. We have to establish the following points:
- An objective evaluation of the sequelae.
- A demonstration of the causality bonds.
- A relation to an anterior state.
- A study of the evolution of the lesions.
- A quantitative evaluation of the injury.

That is why we suggest a guide for the otoneurological approach to patients suffering from whiplash injury [1-3].

Equilibrium Tests

The following tests should be included:
1. Oculomotricity study
   - Saccadic tests

Maître de Conférences Université de Liège, Rue de Bruxelles 21 - B-4800 Verviers, Tel. 87-221760, Fax 87-224608

- Pursuit tests
- Optokinetic tests
2. Vestibulo-ocular reflex study
   - Spontaneous nystagmus
   - Position and positioning nystagmus
   - Rotatory tests
   - Caloric tests
3. Posture tests
4. Gait tests
5. Various
   - Vegetative disturbance analysis
   - Cortico-equilibrium tests

Audiological Tests

These include:
1. Tonal audiometry
2. Supra-threshold audiometry
3. Speech audiometry
4. Tests for malignering
5. Evoked potentials
   - BERA
   - Middle latency
   - Cortical audiometry
6. Tympanogram and stapedius reflex
7. Acoustic otoemission

Other Cranial Nerve Examinations

The following tests should be performed:
1. Gustometry
2. Olfactometry
3. Facial nerve testing

Conclusion

As we have written in the report of the first EUFOS (European United Federation of Otorhinolaringological Societies) meeting [4], there is a great discordance not only between the members of the medical profession but also between the laws and rules concerning disability throughout Europe.

We hope that in the near future a European disability scale will be clearly defined. The proposal for a standard battery test will be the first step in the right direction.

References

1. Boniver R (1994) European medico-legal aspects of vertigo. Neurotology Newsletter 1:78-83
2. Cesarani A, Alpini D (1992) Aspetti medico-legali di disturbi dell'equilibrio. Bi & Gi Ed, Verona
3. Boniver R, Norré M (1986) Expertise médicale en oto-rhino-laryngologie. Recommandations. Acta ORL Belgica 40:907-915
4. Boniver R, Norré M (1988) Medico-Legal in ENT. Meeting of the first european conference of the European Society of Otorhinolaryngology, Paris, Acta ORL Belgica 42:723-770

PART 4

TREATMENT

Pharmacological Treatment of Whiplash Injury

E. A. Pallestrini, E. Castello and G. Garaventa

Introduction

Whiplash injury is a very common cause of vertigo and dizziness especially in the developed countries where this pathology is often related to the increasing number of traffic accidents. The most frequent cause of neck injury is the rear end automobile collision. In this case one of the occupants is thrown into the windshield; this may compress and hyperextend or hyperflex the neck depending on which part of the head strikes the windshield and the position of the neck at impact.

The physiopathological mechanisms of this kind of injury can be explained from the effect of forces applied to the head and the neck during the collision. In the first phase the force applied to the rear end of the car during the collision results in a forward acceleration of the body while the head is pushed backwards from inertial forces causing a cervical hyperextension. In the second phase, which always occurs because of the effect of inertial forces, the head is pushed forward with subsequent hyperflexion of the neck. The whole duration of these phases is about 20 ms. This is the reason for the lack of activation of neck neuromuscular protective reflexes, whose latency is about 50 ms. During neck hyperextension the elongation of cervical rachidian tissues may even reach 5 cm [12-15].

Neck lesions may involve bone and muscle-tendinous structures, intervertebral disks, cervical blood vessels (especially the vertebral arteries), spinal nerve roots, esophagus laryngeal nerves, spinal cord and brainstem.

Head damage can involve skull, CNS structures, peripheral vestibular end organs, cranial nerves, cochlea, etc.

Experimental studies have shown a correlation between the degree of neck hyperextension and the severity of injuries produced [14]. Lesser injuries are due to anterior neck muscle haemorrhages and muscle tears, while more severe injuries are due to anterior longitudinal ligament rupture, disc separation and brain contusion. Regarding this last case (in animal models), elec-

I Divisione O.R.L., Dipartimento Regionale Testa Collo, Ospedale San Martino, Genova, Italy

troencephalographic monitoring showed brain activity decreasing immediately following injury [35].

Symptoms of whiplash injuries are correlated to the severity and anatomical localization of the lesions. Most of them emanate from the muscoloskeletal structures of the neck, while others from the CNS or nerves, eyes, ears, jaw, blood vessels and tracheo-esophageal structures.

The vestibular system is frequently involved in whiplash injuries; lesions may involve labyrinth and central vestibular organs and pathways and can be detected neurootologically, as demonstrated through electronystagmographic findings [28].

Three lesion levels of vestibular system can be distinguished: (1) labyrinth and organ damage; (2) central vestibular and oculomotor system damage; (3) both involvement of the peripheral and central vestibular system.

The evolution of symptoms and vestibular compensation processess are related to the site of the lesions and to the age of the patients. In peripheral vestibular syndromes, compensation phenomena are more effective than in central lesions, in which structures subject to compensation processes are involved in the damage.

In the elderly the evolution of post-traumatic vestibular disorders differs significantly from aging alone and are related to less efficient CNS plasticity with respect to compensation and functional reorganization after the damage. This is principally due to the physiological diminuition of neurotransmitters that are important for the processes that start and modulate compensation.

Table 1 reports the classification of post-traumatic vertigo (from [2], modified).

Pharmacological treatment of vertigo due to whiplash injury should be principally programmed on the basis of otoneurological findings, which al-

Table 1. Causes of post-traumatic vertigo

Damage site	Lesions	Physiopathology
Labyrinth	Labyrinthine lesions, temporal bone fractures, concussive trauma, haemorraggia	
	Maculae - semicircular canals	Otholitic deplacement
	Perilymphatic fistula	Round - oval window rupture
Vestibular nerve	Axomotmesis neurotmesis	Concussion - hemorrhage
Brainstem cerebellum	Concussion hemorrhage ischemia	Neurotransmitter release
Cervical rachis	Whiplash syndrome	Vascular-proprioceptive

low precise topodiagnosis of vestibular system lesions, and on the age of the patient [19-21].

In the child, pharmacological treatment of vestibular post-traumatic disorders is essentially symptomatic for the early and efficient development of compensatory mechanisms. The main aspects of treatment are related essentially to the dosages and the frequency and duration of drug administration for each case. The choice of substance is based on the clinical experience of the physician and on knowledge of the pharmacological characteristics of the different categories of drugs [3, 4, 13, 16].

In the elderly, pharmacological treatment of post-traumatic vertigo shows particular aspects linked to the aging processes. Several factor such as relative enhancement of fat tissue, the reduction of body mass, decreased hepatic and kidney functions and the diminution of serum albumin influence drug pharmacokinetic properties (absorbency, tissue distribution, metabolism, sensibility and clearance).

We can distinguish therapies for isolated peripheral lesions, central lesions or both.

Peripheral Lesions

Benign Positional Vertigo (BPV)

Benign positional vertigo (Cupulolithiasis) is one of the most frequent vestibular manifestation of whiplash injury.

Pharmacological treatment of paroxysmal vertigo due to BPV secondary to whiplash injury is not etiological, but symptomatic drugs and physiotherapy are the main treatment of these disorders.

Symptomatic therapy involves vestibular-suppressor and antiemetic drugs.

Among the vestibular-suppressor drugs, the antihistamines, phenothiazines and benzodiazepines are the most widely used.

Antihistaminic drugs (dimenhydrinate, flunarizine, cinnarizine, hydroxyzine, betahistine, astemizole) act on the synapses between the first and the second neurons, on the reticular formation, on vestibular dopaminergic pathways and on H1 receptors. The pharmacological effect is vestibule-suppressive with inhibition of positional nystagmus [9].

Phenothiazines (promethazine, thiethylperazine, prochlorperazine) are very effective in decreasing acute vertiginous symptoms and vegetative side effects. Pharmacological effects on the vestibular system are the inhibition of peripheral cholinergic inputs; inhibition of H1 receptors in vestibular nuclei and an effect on the bulbar chemoreceptor trigger zone. These drugs decrease vestibular and opticokinetic nystagmus. Phenothiazines have important side effects on the extra pyramidal system, on pressure control mechanisms and on prolactin secretion. For these reasons phenothiazines should be administrated carefully especially in the elderly.

Scopolamine shows strong anticholinergic activity on brainstem, reticular formation and vestibular nuclei. This drug cannot be used in patients suffering from glaucoma, prostatic hypertrophy and heart diseases.

Benzodiazepines (diazepam, lorazepam, etc.) enhance GABA-ergic inhibitory properties of vestibulo-cerebellum on vestibular nuclei and activate internuclear inhibitory pathways. These drugs have inhibitory effects on breathing and blood circulation and worsen the quality of compensation [33].

Pharmacological therapy can be employed during rehabilitative treatment of post-traumatic cupulolithiasis [24]. The aim of drug treatment is to reduce hypertonic contracture of muscles of the neck to facilitate physiotherapeutic treatment and to improve the efficacy of such therapy. *Muscle relaxant substances* can be divided into: (1) drugs active on CNS (mephenesin, carysoprol); (2) drugs with spinal actions (baclofen); (3) drugs active on the muscular system (dantrolene); (4) drugs active on the different systems (thiocolchicoside).

Baclofen has other pharmacological effects on vestibulo-cerebellum (GABA-ergic action) and is employed in the treatment of periodic alternate nystagmus that arises from lesions of lower brainstem. *β-Blockers* reduce muscular hypertonicity of cervical spine and they can be employed as well as proper muscle relaxant drugs. *Propanolol* has been successfully employed in the treatment of whiplash injury-related vertigo. This drug reduces hypertonicity of spinal muscles lowering the discharge frequency of neuromuscular fusicellular endings, with a subsequent diminution of cervical pain [11].

Other Labyrinthine Lesions

Damage to the vestibular apparatus due to whiplash injuries produces acute symptoms, which gradually improve as central compensation occurs. After unilateral vestibular lesions a new sensorineural organization take place with shunts of proprioceptive and visual information toward the side affected. These neuronal processes are enhanced with respect to imbalance perception and on this pharmacotheraphy of vertigo is based.

The aim of the pharmacological strategy in peripheral vestibular lesions however is to improve CNS restorage mechanisms; for this reasons vestibulo-suppressive drugs, even if effective in reducing vertigo and imbalance, worsen the CNS compensation and should be administered only in the first stage of the disease. On the other hand with the employment of CNS excitatory drugs or drugs with decompensating effects during rehabilitative training, compensation processes will be stimulated with acceleration of healing.

At the early stage of disease the administration of cholinergic, adrenergic and GABA-ergic drugs, through a decompensating action improving the perception of vestibular imbalance, will stimulate and accelerate CNS compensatory processes. Afterward when the reorganisation processes have been started and vestibular symptoms are improved, CNS modulator drugs and neuroactive drugs to enhance compensation should be used.

In chronic vertigo where compensation phenomena are incomplete cycles of decompensating drugs should be given to stimulate the CNS to enhance compensation processes (pharmacological training) [18].

In the elderly where CNS reorganisation after vestibular damage is less effective, drugs with positive effects on compensation, as well as haemorrheologic and neuroactive drugs should be used. Careful pharmacological training with decompensating drugs associated with haemorrheologic and neuroactive drugs should be started in chronic peripheral vertigo. Drugs which increase CNS neurotransmitter storage will be also useful in these patients [23].

Symptomatic treatment of vertigo (antihistamines, benzodiazepines, phenothiazines, scopolamine) is helpful in the beginning and can be associated with muscle relaxant substances.

Antihistaminics are the most used drugs in acute labyrinthine lesions. These drugs show strong anti-cholinergic properties and act on the synapses between the I and II neuron and activating reticular formation on dopaminergic pathways and on H1 receptors for their main pharmacological effects on the peripheral vestibular system. The pharmacological result is a vestibulo-suppressive action with inhibition of spontaneous and evoked nystagmus.

Betahistine interferes with the diamine oxidase prolonging histamine action; it has a moderate agonist activity on H1 receptors and a strong activity as an H3 antagonist. Betahistine inhibits neurons of the lateral vestibular nuclei [32] and increases the basilar and cochlear flow in animal models. Betahistine has vasodilatative effects on stria vascularis, spiral ligament and on vertebro-basilar circulation [31]. Betahistine improves microcirculatory flow of the inner ear and central vestibular system and this can explain the positive effects in the treatment of Meniere's disease and in paroxysmal peripheral vertigo of vascular origin. Betahistine has been successfully employed in the preventive treatment of these diseases and this was interpreted as a modulating effect on cerebral and labyrinthine circulation.

Oosterveld (1984) found a diminution of evoked nystagmus after betahistine uptake.

Astemizole has a strong inhibitory action on vertigo and nystagmus and it is interesting from a clinical point of view because it crosses the blood-cerebrospinal-encephalic barrier only in a minimal concentration; for this reason this drug has very low sedative effects and therefore its main action is on the peripheral vestibular system. Astemizole would be not effective in treating CNS disorders and vascular vertigo.

Among drugs which enhance compensation processes, the *amphetamines*, *ginkgo biloba* and *calcium antagonists* are the most used. Amphetamines theoretically could be employed in the treatment of peripheral vestibular lesions based on their positive effects on compensation processes. Their use is limited because of significant side effects. Pemoline and fipexide belong to this category of drugs and are particularly interesting for their limited side effects; pemoline affects dopamine turnover and has few peripheral effects; fipexide affects the reticular formation and shows dopamimetic effects.

Ginkgo biloba enhances postural and locomotor balance and oculomotor function recovery in experimental unilateral vestibular lesions [17, 30].

Cinnarizine and *Flunarizine* selectively block calcium entry into peripheral vestibular system cells (especially cristae cells); both these drugs show antihistaminic and anti-cholinergic activities. In the peripheral vestibular system calcium antagonists modulate neurotransmitter release. Flunarizine interferes in ACh release and enhances compensation processes [22]. In elderly patients these drugs should be administered carefully for its Parkinson's like effects after prolonged treatment [34, 36].

Treatment of perilymphatic fistula is essentially surgical while vestibulo-suppressive drugs may be used to reduce vertigo and vegetative effects.

Medical treatment of post-traumatic lesions of the eighth cranial nerve often is not effective and therapy should follow the rules of unilateral vestibular lesion management.

Central Lesions

Vestibular central system can be involved in whiplash injuries. Physiopathological mechanisms include: (1) direct concussive damage which can impair brainstem and cerebral structures or (2) damage of blood vessels which irritate the vestibular system.

In central lesions the compensatory processes are less efficacious in repairing the damage to the CNS site where compensation phenomena are located. Pharmacological treatment in these cases is indicated to restore and activate CNS functions acting on vestibular neurotransmitters and improving blood circulation. Neuroactive drugs are employed for their actions on CNS neurotransmitters while vasoactive substances improving blood macro- and microcirculation enhance CNS metabolism.

Neuroactive substances can be classified as drugs not specifically acting on vestibular neurotransmitters and drugs specifically acting on vestibular neurotransmitters (Tables 2, 3).

Among neuroactive drugs not specifically active on vestibular neurotransmitters, *citicoline* has dopaminergic and serotonergic activities and reduces platelet aggregatability. *Deanol* and *oxiracetam* have cholinergic action; *pi-*

Table 2. Neuroactive drugs not specifically acting on vestibular neurotransmitters

Metabolic enhancers	Citicoline deanol, piracetam, oxiracetam, ginkgo biloba, protirelin, L-acetylcarnitine
Neuronotrophics	Gangliosides
Excitants	Amphetamines, fipexide, pemoline
Antidepressants	Tricycles IMAO, sulpiride
Anticonvulsants	Carbamazepine
Myorelaxants	Baclofen
β-blockers	

Table 3. Neuroactive drugs specifically acting on vestibular neurotransmitters

Antihistamines	Flunarizine, cinnarizine, hydroxyzine astemizole, betahistine diphenhydramine dymenhydrinate
Phenothiazinies	Promethazine, thiethylperazine, procloroperazine
Benzodiazepines	
Scopolamine	

racetam, a GABA derivative, has strong dopaminergic and mild GABA-ergic activities and improves cerebral ATP synthesis; this drug accelerates compensation phenomena and is well indicated in brainstem disinhibition vertigo [5] and in post-traumatic vestibular lesions [10]. Ginkgo biloba increases cerebral ATP synthesis, normalizes oxygen consumption and has antiaggregating and haemorrheologic properties. *Protirelin* is a TRH derivative; this drug main effect is on the cholinergic neurotransmitter system and shows secondary effects on dopaminergic, noradrenergic and serotonergic systems.

Gangliosides seem to stimulate axonal sprouting and neosynaptogenesis. Among the amphetamines *pemoline* and *fipexide* work on dopamine turnover and have few peripheral effects. In animals these drugs enhance memory and the cognitive processes while in human these effects are secondary. These drugs increase the arousal condition and favour incoming compensation.

Phenothiazines, benzodiazepines and scopolamine belong to the category of neuroactive drugs specifically active on vestibular neurotransmitters.

Phenothiazines, for their peripheral effects, are not employed in central vestibular system lesions arising from whiplash injuries.

Benzodiazepines (diazepam, lorazepam, alprazolam) present a GABA-ergic activity enhancing inhibitory cerebello-vestibular pathways and activating internuclear inhibitory pathways. They are also active on glycinergic pathways, on substantia nigra, on the limbic system and on cholinergic activatory reticular formation. The final effect is the inhibition of the vestibulo-oculomotor reflex and nystagmus. Benzodiazepines have inhibitory effects on breathing and blood circulation and for these reasons should be carefully administered in elderly patients.

Scopolamine has an anti-cholinergic activity and works particularly on brainstem pathways, on reticular formation and vestibular nuclei. This drug improves vertiginous symptoms obtained experimentally and inhibits caloric and opto-kinetic nystagmus but has no effect on nystagmus evoked by rotatory stimulations [27, 29].

Scopolamine has been successfully employed in post-traumatic vertigo with brainstem involvement [6].

Frequently, in whiplash injuries with involvement of CNS, blood vessels of the brainstem, spinal cord and cervical rachis are damaged and in these cases *vasoactive and antiaggregating drugs* can be used alone or in association with other substances such as neuroactives, muscle relaxant substances, etc.

The employment of pure vasodilatative drugs such as papaverine and derivatives has nowadays been replaced by the use of safer and more efficacious substances like haemorrheologics and calcium antagonists. Pure vasodilatative drugs can cause "steal-like" phenomena, hypotension and other important side effects especially in older patients. In this category of drugs interesting substances are *cyclandelate* and *naphthylrophurile*, mandelic derivatives having structural analogies to papaverine. Their main pharmacological property is the inhibition of phosphodiesterase and the increment of intracellular c-AMP; the result is an arteriolar vasodilatation. Thereafter these drugs show calcium antagonist effects with a haemorrheologic effect due to platelet aggregation.

Among α-blockers *dihydroergotoxine*, an alkaloid derivative, has vascular and metabolic activities enhancing α-adrenoceptor blocking activity. Dihydroergotoxine also has a dopaminergic activity and inhibits the specific cerebral phosphodiesterase response in c-AMP metabolism. Their use is however limited to selected cases.

Nicergoline is an ergot derivative with actions on dopamine turnover, on cerebral blood flow and on cerebral glucose consumption; this drug enhances neurotransmitter restorage and for this reason its employment seems to be interesting in post-traumatic vertigo of central origin especially in the elderly.

Drugs active on the microcirculatory system have been found to have multiple actions on the neurotransmitter system, on cerebral flow and cerebral metabolism with limited side effects. Among these substances *buflomedil* has α-blocking, antiaggregant and haemorrheologic properties and a calcium antagonist effect. This drug acts to diminish cerebral oxygen consumption [7].

Pentoxifylline has different pharmacological properties; the main one is the improvement of erythrocyte deformability (through an ATP improvement) and the diminution of blood viscosity (through a diminution of fibrinogen). This drug reduces platelet aggregation by acting on membrane phosphodiesterases, reducing thromboxane synthesis and improving at the same time the synthesis of prostacycline. Pentoxifylline reduces platelet adhesiveness to the vessel wall and results in a delayed thrombogenic action.

Among calcium antagonists *nimodipine* improves DOPA action inhibiting ACh, GABA and glutamate; this drug has a strong cerebral vasodilatative effect without a steal effect and without pressure modifications. Its pharmacological action seems to be prevalently directed to ward small vessels improving the cerebral flow. *Nicardipine* is usually useful in the treatment of arterial hypertension and in angina; this drug has a cerebral vasodilatative action and improves the flow and oxygen liberation. *Cinnarizine* has vasodilatatory, antihistamine and anticholinergic effects inhibiting central vestibular system activities. Cinnarizine shows a better effect in reducing nystagmus duration than betahistine.

The main CNS action of flunarizine, difluorinate derivative of cinnarizine, is blocking Ca^{2+} blocking entry into cells during hypoxia. Flunarizine has a stronger and more prolonged action than cinnarizine (Oosterveld 1974).

Boniver found a significant reduction in the duration of the angular velocity of nystagmus in patients suffering from vertigo of vascular origin [1]. Hofferberth (1980) attested to a normalisation of the electronystagmographic parameters in a high percentage of cases after 8 weeks of treatment with flunarizine (20 mg/day). Pfaltz and Aoyagi [26] organised a comparative study on the therapeutic efficacy of flunarizine, betahistine and diethylperazine in vertigo of vascular origin; the authors found a significant diminution of gain (the most significant parameter for pharmacological effects on vestibular-oculomotor reflex) in the group treated with flunarizine. Similar results were obtained by Staessen (1977) on a group of 300 patients.

Muller and Blum (1981), in a double blind study, found a more significant improvement of electronystagmographic findings in patients treated with flunarizine compared to those treated with vincamine.

Elbaz found, in vertigo due to vertebro-basilar insufficiency, a more therapeutic effect of flunarizine than of betahistine [8].

In animals Weinten and Herder [34] found an effect of flunarizine on atherogenic substances.

Verapamil shows dilatory effect on vessels causing a total peripheral low with respect to resistance. The pharmacological mechanism is the inhibition of vessel contractility. *Gallopamil* inhibits in a reversible way calcium flow through the fibrocellular smooth muscle cell wall inducing a vasodilatatory effect both in arteries and veins.

New generations of antiaggregating drugs have several actions on the blood vessel wall and on coagulative processes without significant side effects [25]. *Ticlodipine* has an antiaggregant effect. It inhibits fibrinogen-platelet linkage, stimulates platelet disaggregation and diminishes erythrocyte aggregation. *Picotamide* inhibits thromboxane A2 synthesis and interactions the thromboxane-A2 receptor. This drug doesn't interfere with endothelial synthesis of prostacycline. *Mesoglicane*, a mixture of heparan-sulphate, dermatan and chondroitin sulphate reduces platelet adhesiveness and has fibrionolytic activity via reactivation of endothelial synthases of plasminogen activator. The drug favours endothelial barrier function and enhances vessel elasticity by its action on the connective tissue component of the vessel wall. *Dipyridamole* has an important activity on platelet aggregation; the main functions are inhibition of platelet phosphodiesterase and endothelial prostacycline synthesis.

Currently, first generation substances (acetylsalicylic acid and heparin) are less often used in the treatment of post-traumatic vertigo due to their side effects.

Acetylsalicylic acid inhibits irreversibly the cyclo-oxygenase enzyme blocking thromboxane (aggregant and vasoconstrictive activities) and prostacycline (anti-aggregant and vasodilatative actions).

Heparin's anticoagulative properties are related to its linkage with antithrombin III protein. Low dose heparin has an antithrombotic action on the vessel wall surface because it is recognized by endothelial cells.

Pharmacological Strategy in Whiplash Injury

Pharmacological treatment of vertigo due to whiplash injuries should be developed on the basis of otoneurologic findings which allow determination of the site of the lesions.

In benign positional vertigo drug treatment should principally support rehabilitative training. Neck pain and muscular stiffness and spasm make difficult vestibular physical treatment in the early stage of the disease; for these reasons, muscle relaxant substances or β-blockers improving muscular spasm allow early rehabilitative training. Propanolol is particularly indicated because of its strong action on cervical pain and on vertigo.

These drugs should be combined with vestibular sedative substances (benzodiazepines, antihistamines, phenothiazines, scopolamine) to improve vertigo and the neurovegetative symptoms, but long term treatment should be avoided due to negative effects on compensation processes and side effects. Vestibular sedative drugs should be employed immediately after head-neck trauma and continued for a few days.

In labyrinthine lesions the preferred drugs are those with positive effects on vestibular compensation. Ginkgo biloba and calcium antagonists have been demonstrated to improve and accelerate compensation phenomena and formation of haemorrheologic substances. Vestibular suppressive drugs would be helpful initially to improve vertigo and neurovegetative phenomena but should be avoided for long treatments.

In post-traumatic vertigo of central origin, pharmacological therapy should be planned based on otoneurological findings and on CNS site lesions. Drugs active on neurotransmitter systems may be employed together with vasoactive substances that improve CNS circulation and metabolism.

In brainstem involvement drugs active on the cholinergic, histaminergic and adrenergic neurotransmitter systems (scopolamine, cinnarizine) are effective in reducing symptoms, but can interfere with compensation processes.

In cases exhibiting lack of cerebello-vestibular control drugs with GABA-ergic actions such as piracetam and benzodiazepines may be employed successfully.

Vasoactive drugs are widely used in post-traumatic vestibular lesions of central origin. This category of substances often shows multiple pharmacological effects on cerebral blood flow (buflomedil, nicergoline), on inner ear microcirculation (pentoxyfylline), on blood vessel walls (nimodipine, nicardipine, verapamil), on platelets and erythrocytes (pentoxyfylline, naphthylrophurile) on CNS metabolism and on neurotransmitter systems (most of them). Their therapeutical efficacy is improved by their lack of negative effects on compensation processes and the possibility of long term treatment.

In the treatment of elderly patients, in whom neurotransmitter levels are decreased, drugs that improve neurotransmitter functions such as nicergoline should be preferred.

References

1. Boniver R (1979) Vertigo particularly of vascular origin, treated with flunarizine. Acta Otolaryngol Bel 33:270-281
2. Brandt T (1991) Vertigo. Its multisensory syndromes. Springer-Verlag, Berlin
3. Bronner G, Gentile A, Conraux C, Collard M (1981) Les modifications des les ENGrafie induites par les drogues actives sur le systeme vestibulo-oculaire central. Rev Oto Neuro Ophtalmol 53:95-110
4. Casani A, Ghilardi B, Fattori B (1992) La terapia delle sindromi vertiginose post-traumatiche. In: Il danno vestibolare nei disturbi cranio-cerebrali, Pistoia, 31 ottobre
5. Claussen CF, Schneider D, Patil NP (1989) The treatment of minocycline induced brainstem vertigo by the combined administration of Piracetam and Ergotoxin. Acta Otolaryngol Stock [Suppl 468]:171-174
6. Childs A (1986) Scopolamine effects in vestibular defensiveness. Arch Phys Med Rehabil 67:554-555

7. Clissold SP, Lynch S, Sorkin EM (1987) Buflomedil Drugs 33:430-460
8. Elbaz P (1988) Flunarizine and Betahistine. Two different therapeutic approaches in vertigo compared in a double bind study Acta Otolaryngol [Suppl 460]:143-148
9. Fischer A (l991) Histamine in the treatment of vertigo. Acta Otolaryngol Stock [Suppl 479]:24-28
10. Futschik D (1991) Therapeutical concepts in post-traumatic vestibular lesions. In: Claussen CF, Kirtane MV (eds) Vertigo, nausea, tinnitus and hypoacusia due to head neck trauma. Elsevier, Amsterdam, p 193
11. Hinoky M (1985) Vertigo due to whiplash injury: a neurologic approach. Acta Otolaryngol [Suppl 419]:9-14
12. Hohl M (1990) Soft tissue neck injuries. A review. Rev Chir Orthop 76 [Suppl 1]:16-25
13. Igarashi M, Oosterveld WJ, Thomsen J, Watanabe I, Rubin W (1983) Medical treatment of vertigo. How valutate its effect? Adv Oto-rhino-Laryngol 30:345-349
14. Macnab I (1964) Acceleration injuries of the cervical spine. J Bone Joint Surg [Am]46:1797-1799
15. Macnab I (1965) Whiplash injuries of the neck. Am Assoc Automotive Med
16. Malavasi Gananca M, Caovilla HH (1994) Treatment of dizziness and vertigo in children. In: Cesarani A, Alpini D (eds). Diagnosi e trattamento dei disturbi dell'equilibrio nell'età evolutiva ed involutiva. Milano, 83-89
17. Malavasi Gananca M, Caovilla HH, Freitas Gananca F, Serafini F (1994) Medical treatment of brainstem and cerebellar equilibrium disturbances: nicergoline and ginkgo biloba. In: Cesarani A, Alpini D (eds). Equilibrium disorders. Brainstem and cerebellar pathology. Springer-Verlag, 176-182
18. Pallestrini EA, Accomando E, Gatti M (1983) La terapia della vertigine nel corso di training vestibolare. Acta Otolaryngol It 3:289-294
19. Pallestrini EA, Accomando E, Borasi F, Garaventa G (1985) Interferenze farmacologiche nello studio dei movimenti oculari di interesse otoneurologico Acta Otolaryngol It 3:289-294
20. Pallestrini EA, Accomando E, Bertoglio C, Gatti M, Garaventa G, Castiglia GC (1984) Il nistagmo da privazione vertebro-basilare. Otorinolaringologia 34:259-271
21. Pallestrini EA, Garaventa G, Accomando E, Borasi F, Maffezzoni E (1985) Aspetti elettronistagmografici dell'insufficienza vertebro-basilare. Boll It Biologia sperimentale 8:1093-1100
22. Pallestrini EA, Garaventa G Bindi G (1990) Nuove acquisizioni nella terapia farmacologica della vertigine. In: X Giornata Italiana di Nistagmografia Clinica, Sorrento
23. Pallestrini EA, Garaventa G, Castello E (1991) Problemi di farmacoterapia della vertigine nell'anziano. In: Cesarani A, Alpini D (eds). Diagnosi e trattamento dei disturbi dell'equilibrio nell'età evolutiva ed involutiva. Milano, 223-236
24. Pallestrini EA, Castello E (1992) La terapia farmacologica della vertigine parossistica benigna. In: XII Giornata italiana di nistagmografia clinica, Viterbo, 99-110
25. Pallestrini EA, Garaventa G, Castello E (1994) Equilibrium disorders. In: Cesarani A, Alpini D (eds) Equilibrium disorders. Springer-Verlag Milano p 183

26. Pfaltz CR, Aoyagi M (1988) Calcium-blockers in the treatment of vestibular disorders. Acta Otolaryngol [Suppl 460]:135-142
27. Pyykko I, Padoan S, Schalen L, Lyttkens L, Magnusson M, Henriksson NG (1985) The effects of TTS-scopolamine, dimenhydrinate, lidocaine and tocainide on motion sickness, vertigo and nystagmus. Aviat Space Environ Med 56:777-782
28. Rubin W (1973) Whiplash with vestibular involvement. Arch Otolaryngol 97:85-87
29. Shojaku H, Watanabe Y, Ito M, Mizukoshi K, Yajima K, Sekiguchi C (1993) Effect of transdermally administred scopolamine on the vestibular system in humans. Acta Otolaryngol, Stock, 504:41-45
30. Smith PF, Darlington CL (1994) Can vestibular compensation be enhanced by drug treatment? A review of recent evidence. J Vestib Res 4:169-179
31. Tomita M, Gotoh F, Sato TT (1978) Comparative responses of the carotid and vertebral arterial system of rhesus monkeys to betahistine. Stroke 9:382-387
32. Uemoto H, Sasa M, Takaori S, Ito J, Matsvoka I (1982) Inhibitory effect of betahistine on polysinaptic neurons in the lateral vestibular nucleus. Arch Otolaryngol 236:229-236
33. Zee DS (1985) Perspective on pharmacotherapy of vertigo. Arch Otolaryngol, Stock, 11:609-612
34. Weinstein DB, Herder JG (1988) The antiatherosclerotic potential of calcium antagonists In: Calcium antagonists in hypertension. Internat Symp Basle, 11-12
35. Wickstrom J, Martinez J, Rodriguez R (1967) Cervical sprain syndrome and experimental acceleration injuries of the head and neck In: The prevention of highway injury. Highway safety Institute Ann Arbor, Michigan
36. Wouters DV, Amery MD, Towse G (1983) Flunarizine in the treatment of vertigo. J Laringol Otol 97:697-704

Whiplash Injury: Orthopaedic and Rehabilitative Approach to Neck Pathology

P. Sibilla, S. Negrini and S. Atanasio

The term whiplash classically has been applied to a variable set of clinical circumstances where a non-severe rear-end collision is involved. Nowadays [73-75] this definition has changed, because this term also includes other types of accidents with different mechanisms: lateral collisions, frontal ones, as well as falls with direct trauma to the head and hypermovement in one direction of the neck. The common point between these different types of pathologic conditions is that this trauma causes a damage to the cervical soft tissues without engagement of bones.

The Quebec Task Force on Whiplash-Associated Disorders (1995) [71-72] adopted the following definition: "Whiplash is an acceleration - deceleration mechanism of energy transfer to the neck. It may result from rearend or side-impact motor vehicle collisions, but can also occur during diving or other mishaps. The impact may result in bony or soft-tissue injuries (whiplash injury), which in turn may lead to a variety of clinical manifestations (whiplash-associated disorders)". We agree with this interpretation [48-50].

The clinical picture is characterised by a large variety of symptoms with a common complaint of neck pain in the vast majority of the patients. Radiographs of the cervical spine are generally normal.

In this chapter we will discuss the orthopaedic and rehabilitative treatment of whiplash, identifying five clinical degrees of pathology and proposing different orthopaedic therapeutic approaches. Then each rehabilitative tool will be discussed, focusing particularly on the restoration of neck tissue functioning [1, 14, 15, 20, 24, 30, 31, 33, 35].

Clinical Picture

In this section we will discuss the general clinical elements that will be presented thoroughly below, where the five degrees of whiplash injuries will be discussed.

Reparto Scoliosi e Patologia Vertebrale, IRCCS, Fondazione Pro-Juventute, Don Carlo Gnocchi, Milan, Italy

The following topics will be covered:
1. Anatomical pathology
2. History
3. Clinical examination
   • Range of movement (RoM)
   • Palpation
   • Neurologic examination
4. Imaging
5. Diagnosis
6. Treatment

Anatomical Pathology

In this section the soft tissues involved will be discussed [2-3]. It is necessary to clarify that studies of real soft tissue involvement do not exist particularly in less important lesions. There are however reasonable proposals based on literature findings.

When the injury occurs, the *ligaments* and *zygapophyseal joints* that are strained and/or disrupted by the accident are the most important soft tissues involved [16, 29], whereas *discs* are less important at the beginning, when the accident is recent. However, they can be the most important pathological elements for the future of the patient. Tears produced in the outer part of the discs when the injury occurred become "loci minoris resistentiae" where bulging, protrusions and/or real herniations can appear. We know that discal lesions are likely to be the most common cervical pathologies in these patients and that they can partially justify the continuation of some symptoms [17, 28].

Muscles heal rapidly with a little rest; *tendons* could be more significantly involved, but they are treated the same way as ligaments and capsules. Conversely, muscles are fundamental in the rehabilitative process [23, 26, 27].

The most dramatic symptoms can begin and remain because of *nervous tissue* involvement. Unfortunately, here is where we know less: medulla, brain, nerve roots, sympathetic plexus can be all involved in different manners justifying the multiform symptoms [18, 19, 52, 53].

History

At the very beginning of the history of a classical whiplash patient there is an accident [54].

Pain

Pain in the neck is the most common problem. At the beginning, pain usually is not precisely localised by the patient and it is increased by any type of motion. Normally it is not confined to the neck, spreading to the head or to one of the upper extremities.

After a few hours to a few days the discomfort in the anterior region of the neck disappears and the patient can localise his problem in one posterior region of the neck and/or in one of the upper limbs much more precisely.

In contrast to what happens in common discal problems, pain is not a very important clue in determining the gravity of the lesion and the pathomechanical characteristics of the injury [8, 10-12, 44, 45].

Motion

In a first degree whiplash active movements are slightly reduced; later they become more blocked. At the beginning, this is usually not a major complaint of the patient, but with time it could become an important problem, particularly if rotations are decreased [4-6].

Daily Life Positions

In all these lesions, beginning with a first degree whiplash and increasing in magnitude, it is impossible to maintain standing and/or sitting positions for long periods. Fatiguability is important and it is due initially to the lesion and to pain, but with time to the muscular weakness developed "ex non uso". The patients usually refer to this as a major complaint [76-77].

Other Symptoms

There can be a variety of other symptoms (described in other chapters of this book) such as headache, dizziness, visual disturbances (i.e. blurred vision or scotomata), eye anomalies (i.e. Horner's syndrome), auditory abnormalities (i.e. buzzing or noises), numbness and/or pins and needles to the extremities, drop attacks, tachycardia, sweat to one upper extremity, etc. [7, 9, 34, 59, 60]

Clinical Examination

First of all it must be premised that it is necessary to handle a whiplash injured neck with a lot of care. This is true particularly in First Aid departments and at the first visit. When the healing process is thought to be advanced enough, it is necessary to stress the structures to understand the way they respond to what they will undergo during daily activities.

The standard orthopaedic examination offers different signs immediately after the injury and in subsequent days [61, 62].

It is very important to observe the patient. Usually the neck is placed in an anomalous position that normally corresponds to a forced placement due to the derangement that occurred. Observation is also important to discover difficulties during gait or problems in the eyes that could lead to an incorrect diagnosis.

Range of Movement

Active Evaluation in Sitting
In this position the RoM is generally reduced all the way around in the early period, but it gradually becomes restrained only in a few painful directions.

The pattern of blocked or free movements usually fully describes the pathomechanics of the injury, which can be in this way completely understood.

It is important to test all the eight basic movements possible in the cervical spine. In fact, using the protraction/retraction movements compared to the flexion/extension ones it is possible to better understand the involvement of the upper or lower cervical spine. Rotations and lateral flexions are asymmetrically involved only in cases of a lateral component during the accident.

Metameric Evaluation
It is very interesting to test also the localised motions of the single cervical vertebrae. This can be done in each direction, but is usually evaluated with a combined movement corresponding to the plane of movement of any zygapophyseal joint. Placing a thumb on the joint tested, with the patient usually seated, and passively moving the head in a very gentle manner in flexion/extension combined with a little bit of rotation and lateral flexion, it is possible to feel the articular movement. In the majority of cases restrictions can be felt at many levels. This test can also be done in the supine position along all axes and planes of movement [13].

Supine Passive Evaluation
This evaluation is important in first and second degree lesions. In third degree whiplash, it is better not to examine the RoM in the supine position because sympathetic symptoms increase as a result of moving the cervical spine in this posture. This doesn't happen immediately after the movements: usually it is felt only regaining the sitting or standing position and sometimes during the night or in the morning either just before or after getting out of bed [21].

Palpation
Palpation is a very important tool in the physical examination of a whiplash injured patient (and always in any other pathologic necks). During this phase of the process of evaluating a patient, the real eyes of the examiner are in the tip of his fingers.

Usually it is better to evaluate bony and ligamentous structures in the supine position, because active structures can in this way be placed at rest. Active structures can usually be palpated better when sitting. It is necessary to know how cervical anatomic components "feel" under your fingers and how normal people feel when you touch these points. Then, it will become possible to understand much more about the patient. It is necessary to stress that muscles must also be thoroughly palpated, searching for localised spasms and/or tender/trigger points.

Neurologic Examination

This is a standard evaluation to reveal central and/or peripheral nervous system damages. It has to be more accurate with increasing magnitude of impairment, but it also must not be neglected in first degree whiplash injuries, where the nervous system is sometime the most involved.

Below, the pertinent most common neurologic complications will be discussed [56, 57].

Other Tests

Other tests could be used, such as an examination of vertebral arteries or an evaluation of a possible thoracic outlet syndrome. Usually these tests are not useful in an acute patient [58].

Imaging and Other Examinations

Roentgenography

Timely and accurate diagnosis of cervical spine injury is essential. A complete cervical spine series will diagnose almost 90% of all cervical spine injuries and consists of a lateral roentgenogram from C1 to the top of T1, an AP roentgenogram, and an open mouth view (odontoid). In patients with large shoulders and/or short neck, it is often difficult to visualize the C7-T1 junction on the lateral film and it may be necessary to apply traction to the arms to pull down the shoulders or obtain a swimmer' s view.

Radiographs of the cervical spine after a whiplash injury are generally normal, except for the possible loss of physiologic cervical lordosis. However several clinical and experimental studies lead to the conclusion that the whiplash phenomenon may include occult injuries. These reports suggest that some patients thought to have normal radiographs following whiplash may well have some injuries which are occult on routine radiographs, for example: interarticular isthmus fractures, with or without lamina fractures, fractured transverse process of C1; facet fractures; rotary subluxation of C1 with respect to the occiput and the axis; Luschka joint fractures.

In these cases further studies are needed to determine the extent of injury: dynamic flexion/extension lateral and oblique roentgenograms; pluridirectional tomography and computerized axial tomography.

The role of dynamic lateral radiographs in an emergency setting remains controversial. These views are useful in alert, cooperative patients without neurologic deficit and a normal spine series who continue to complain of neck pain. In this setting a positive flexion/extension study has obvious clinical implications, but a negative roentgenogram does not rule out an acute flexion distraction injury. Patients with acute cervical spine subluxation may have muscle spasm which masks cervical instability for up to 2-3 weeks [55].

Therefore, despite a negative study, for any patient in whom the index of suspicion is high enough to obtain flexion/extension roentgenogram, immobilisation in a rigid orthosis and follow up roentgenogram in 2-3 weeks is recommended.

Oblique radiographs in patients with flexion distraction injuries can be useful in the diagnosis of facet fractures. Obviously they should be obtained by angling the radiograph beam and not rotating the patient's head.

Pluridirectional tomography appears to be particularly advantageous in patients with injuries involving the facets. Computerized tomography appears to add the most additional information in patients with laminar and posterior element fractures and C1 fractures [63, 64].

Static or dynamic flexion/extension lateral plain and AP roentgenogram can show subluxation of cervical vertebrae. Subluxation of the posterior cervical facet joints is caused by a partial disruption of the articular capsule and possibly the intervening intervertebral disc which allows anterior translation of the cephalad vertebra on the more caudad vertebra.

In unilateral dislocation on a lateral plain roentgenogram the cephalad vertebra may appear translated up to 25% of the width of the caudad vertebral body with splaying apart of the posterior spinous processes: the rotational deformity allows visualisation of both facet joints on the lateral roentgenogram (normally superimposed), the so-called bow tie sign. On the AP roentgenogram the spinous processes may be rotated with widening of the interspinous distance.

With bilateral dislocations, both inferior articular processes of the cephalad vertebra dislocate anterior to the superior processes of the caudad vertebra: This results in approximately 50% anterior translation of the superior vertebral body on the inferior vertebral body. There is no rotational deformity (absent bow tie sign) on roentgenographic evaluation and clinically the patient's head is held in the mid-line.

168

It is also very important not to neglect the first part of the thoracic spine, because is not rare to also see vertebral bodies fracture in T1 to T4. In fact, these vertebra are functionally ascribed to the cervical spine by many authors.

Finally, the lower back must not be forgotten, because is not rare that accident can involve this part of the body as well [65-67].

Magnetic Resonance Imaging

This is the choice imaging exam for cervical spine when radiographs show pathologic findings or the clinical examination demonstrated signs suggestive of medullar involvement. The choice depends on the ability to show soft tissues and particularly nervous structures better then CT. The inferior sensibility to disc herniation (MRI "slices" have a thickness of 4-5 mm and TC "slices" can achieve to 1 mm) is not so important at this level of the spine.

Other Examinations

These can include electronystagmography, an echo Doppler to evaluate arterial flow, stabilometry, craniocorpography. These exams are not thoroughly discussed here because they are not completely pertinent to this chapter [68, 69].

First Degree Whiplash

Anatomical Pathology

First degree whiplash is a simple strain of the cervical spine ligaments. The zygapophyseal joints do not show severe lesions although they have been stressed in distraction and compression according to the mechanism of injury. In the outer part of the discs, tears can appear that can justify tardy painful syndromes due to discal protrusions. The muscles are stretched, usually without lesions of their bodies and/or their tendons. An involvement of sympathetic plexus or nerve roots is seldom [70].

History

The pain is not very accentuated, and is usually local, but sometimes there are irradiations to head and/or shoulders. If trigger points appear, there can be irradiation to upper extremities, but these are not due to nerve root involvement.

Symptoms usually are increased by active movements and by prolonged periods of standing and/or sitting. Sympathetic symptoms are rare, but sometimes difficult to treat.

Clinical Examination

If there has been a lateral impact and/or the head of the patient was rotated when the accident occurred, there can be a torticollis, usually with the head away from the pain.

Range of Movement. Usually the cervical spine is relatively mobile. Movements are painful in any direction at the last degrees of the range of movement, the most involved are extension and particularly retraction, many times flexion is free. If there is a lateral component, rotation and lateral flexion are more painful on one side than the other. It's important here to remember that rotation tests better assess the upper cervical spine (occiput-C2) while lateral flexion assesses the medial and inferior segments.

Testing each articular level it is usually possible to find some joints that are more involved. This evaluation is fully compatible with the mechanism of the injury: upper spine if protrusion was prevalent, C5-C6 if flexion/extension was more important, symmetry if only sagittal movements occurred, asymmetry sometimes with differences between lower and upper cervical spine if a lateral component was present.

It is possible to verify RoM also in the supine position, where there are not many differences apart from a trivial increase in the RoM.

Palpation. Muscles are not very painful. A light contracture is present, sometimes only in a few fibres, occasionally trigger points are detectable.

Examining the zygapophyseal joints it is possible to "feel" their involvement as shown by the RoM segmental evaluation. Also the lateral apophysis can be painful [51].

Neurologic examination. It is usually normal.

Imaging

Sometimes a reduction of cervical lordosis appears. This is not the most important finding, because many times it is only a false positive. The clinical examination allows a definite evaluation. Localised inversion of the curve is much more important, as rigidity is limited to a few segments. It is important to recall here that these can come from the daily life activities of the patient, and not from the injury. This is related to age, meaning that it is more likely in the third decade of life than in the second.

Fractures and dislocation must be searched and excluded, but are not pertinent to this clinical picture.

Diagnosis

There is not a real boundary between first and second degree whiplash: they describe a continuum in which the first degree represents the less important clinical lesion and the second degree represents an important clinical picture, with little movement, significant contracture and frequent irradiation of pain.

Treatment

A soft collar must be prescribed for 20 days, because it is necessary to let the ligaments heal. This happens in 18 days normally [32]. The soft collar permits a little protected motion inside. It is not possible to move the cervical spine more than at the beginning of the RoM, but this motion is not only allowable, it is also advisable. In fact it is known that the ligaments heal along the force lines of the movement, if this is permitted, if it is not, the ligamentous tissue repairs in a perturbed fashion.

Rehabilitation can begin after the collar is no longer needed [22, 36, 46, 47].

Whiplash: Second Degree

Anatomical Pathology

Second degree whiplash is a real strain of the ligaments and capsules of the zygapophyseal joints. These do not show dislocations: the capsular involvement depends on their distraction, sometimes internal derangement can be demonstrated. Disc lesions can be protrusions or bulging. The muscles are overstretched, sometimes without lesions of the body: these are more likely to involve tendons at their insertions. There is usually an involvement of the sympathetic plexus. The medulla can be slightly stretched, and sometimes nerve roots are involved too.

History

Pain is local with irradiations to head and/or shoulders. Irradiation to upper extremities is common, rarely due to nerve root lesions. Active movements are sometimes impossible, in most cases they are possible only to a minor degree. Vertigo, dizziness, nausea, vomit, scotomata, and photophobia are common. Sometimes drop attacks can appear too.

Clinical Examination

Usually patients present with a fixed position, fully compatible with the mechanism of injury, including both impact and head position.

Range of Movement. The cervical spine is relatively blocked. Movements are painful in any direction at the very beginning of the RoM: many times the flexion is less involved and the most involved are rotations. The more blocked movements permit one to understand how the accident happened.

To test the more blocked articular levels is usually not useful nor possible, because all of the cervical spine is involved.

The RoM in the supine position is usually a little bit less obstructed.

Palpation. Muscles are painful, usually more at their insertions. An important muscular contracture is present, usually in trapezium, sternocleidomastoid and elevator scapulae. Trigger points in the same muscles are usually detectable.

Examining the zygapophyseal joints it is possible to "feel" their involvement which, at this stage, is normally very important and bilateral, depending on the mechanics of injury. The lateral apophyses are usually painful.

Neurologic Examination. There can be weakness, sensory impairment and/or reflex alterations. These have to be monolateral and monoradicular, otherwise it is necessary to evaluate more thoroughly the lower extremities and the other neurologic functions to investigate a possible medullar or central involvement (rare in second degree whiplash).

Imaging

Reduction of cervical lordosis, localised inversion of the curve or rigidity of a few segments are more likely in this case.

Diagnosis

As was described above, between second and third degree whiplash the differences are only clinical: in third degree usually movements are completely blocked due to the pain, which is more intense and irradiated compared to a second degree lesion. Also sympathetic symptoms are more pronounced.

Treatment

A soft collar with good containment (this means that it allows less movement), or an hard collar must be prescribed for 20 days. It is necessary to pay particular attention to sustaining the cervical spine without distracting/elongating it. It is also very important not to keep the cervical spine in an incorrect position: usually patients with these collars are followed by a technician and not by a physician and this is a mistake. It is important not to hold the patient in protrusion, because this can be exactly the position in which the lesion occurred, but to restrain movements keeping a correct position. If the head is maintained in a protracted position, as long as the patient is sustained he feels well, but when the collar is removed his symptoms return, often worsened exactly by the collar. Rehabilitation must begin after removing the collar. The process must be gradual and determined by the physiotherapist (according to the physician's prescription) on the basis of the gradual training of muscles [23, 37, 38].

Whiplash: Third Degree

Anatomical Pathology

Third degree whiplash is a serious strain of the ligaments that are partially split. Zygapophyseal joints in this case too do not show dislocations: there is only capsular distraction and sometimes internal derangements can be demonstrated. Disc lesions can reach real herniation. Muscles are overstretched, sometimes without lesions of the body but always of tendons at their insertions. There is an important involvement of sympathetic plexus. Medulla can be stretched, and nerve roots usually are involved too.

History

Pain is always irradiated to head and/or shoulders and many times to upper extremities due to nerve root lesions. Active movements are impossible and when the patient is asked to move the neck he only moves his eyes

Vertigo, dizziness, nausea, vomit, scotomata, photophobia and drop attacks are present in most patients.

Sometimes there is tachycardia, pins and needles to both upper and lower extremities (one or both sides), strength or sensory deficits, eye alterations, and sweating to one upper extremity, revealing significant lesions to nervous structures.

Clinical Examination

The patient presents in a fixed position that in this case too is normally a clue to the mechanism of the injury.

Range of Movement. The cervical spine is completely blocked. Active and passive movements are impossible in any direction, although sometimes a little bit of motion appears offering a clue as to how the accident happened.

It is important to be very cautious when testing RoM in the supine position in these patients.

Palpation. Muscles are painful and very contracted but palpation at this stage is not very useful, due to the obvious clinical picture [39-41].

Neurologic Examination. This exam is very important at this stage, and central signs must be very thoroughly examined, because as reported in the literature there may also be encephalic involvements. Nerve root signs are not rare.

Many times it is necessary to investigate these patients using a variety of instruments.

Imaging

In these patients definite radiographic signs are still absent, differentiating third degree from fourth degree whiplash. This is why it is very important to completely and exhaustively evaluate the radiographs.

Diagnosis

Between third and fourth degree whiplash there is a definite boundary: a radiographically evident lesion with subdislocation of zygapophyseal joints.

Treatment

An hard collar must be prescribed for 25-30 days. In these cases it is important to offer a support to both chin and occiput. Many times it is also necessary to extend anteriorly to the sternum, blocking in this way the possibility of moving the head anteriorly or maintaining an incorrect position. Obviously not distracting/elongating the cervical spine, nor keeping an incorrect position is crucial here. Rehabilitation must begin after removing the collar and must be very gradual. The collar must be removed gradually over 15-30 days, always determined by the physiotherapist according to the physician's prescription and closely monitoring training of the muscles [78, 79].

Whiplash: Fourth Degree

Anatomical Pathology

Fourth degree whiplash is a condition in which the mechanical stability of the cervical spine has been compromised. There is a capsular disruption of zygapophyseal joints combined with a ligamentous strain that allows pathological movements between vertebral bodies. In this case too disc lesions such as definite herniation are common. Neurological lesions can include all of what has been described above together with a possible direct compression of nerve structures. A medullar damage can be suspected, but sometimes it appears only later rather than immediately after the injury occurred.

History

Pain is particularly important and does not respond to treatments. Active movements are impossible. All neurological symptoms mentioned above can be presented by the patient.

Clinical Examination

There are not important differences from what has been mentioned regarding third degree whiplash.

Imaging

In these patients there is a subdislocation of one or more articular processes.

This can be seen as an anomalous motion of one vertebral body with respect to the other in dynamic radiographs or as an anomalous monolateral opening of the articular zygapophyseal space. Sometimes the vertebral malalignement can be seen also in plain lateral radiographs. In some cases it is important to also take a lateral dynamic radiographic exam to investigate anomalous motions comparing the two exposures in lateral flexion.

Diagnosis

Between fourth and fifth degree whiplash there is another definite boundary: a complete articular dislocation [42, 43].

Treatment

A Minerva collar in Articast (less heavy than one in simple cast) has to be prescribed for as along as 30-40 days, assuring in this way a complete blockage for a period long enough to permit stabilisation. If this does not occur, it is necessary to stabilise the cervical spine surgically.

The rehabilitation process must be as presented above.

Whiplash: Fifth Degree

This lesion is not completely pertinent to our work. It is very rare, it has a dramatic clinical picture and it is characterised by dislocation of one or more articular processes or by bony fractures.

The risks are very high and it is necessary to act surgically to reduce the lesion with an anterior or posterior fusion.

Discussion of the Classification

In the literature there has been a great heterogeneity of classifications. The Quebec Task Force on Whiplash-Associated Disorders' proposal represents a milestone for both clinicians and researchers. This classification is summarised in Table 1. To better compare this classification with the one we have proposed, we present, in Table 2, other clinical and pathological specifications proposed by the Quebec Task Force on Whiplash-Associated Disorders and, in Table 3, a summary of our classification.

It must be said that we proposed our classification during the S. Margherita Meeting in January 28, 1995, before the appearance in the literature of the

Quebec Task Force classification [71]. The two are surprisingly similar, but ours is more pertinent to our way of treatment and is derived from a more practical, clinical point of view. The Quebec Task Force classification is designed to better compare the literature results about different types of patients

Table 1. Clinical classification on whiplash-associated disorders proposed by the Quebec Task Force (1995) [71]

Grade	Clinical presentation [a]
0	No complaints about the neck No physical sign(s)
I	Neck complaint of pain, stiffness, or tenderness No physical sign(s)
II	Neck complaint and Musculoskeletal sign(s): decreased range of motion and point tenderness
III	Neck complaint and Neurological sign(s): decreased or absent deep tendon reflexes, weakness, and sensory deficits
IV	Neck complaint and Fracture or dislocation

[a] Symptoms and disorders that can be manifest in all grades include deafness, dizziness, tinnitus, headache, memory loss, dysphagia, and temporomandibular joint pain. Grades I-II are the limits of terms of reference of the Quebec Task Force on Whiplash-Associated Disorders [71]

Table 2. Clinical spectrum of whiplash-associated disorders as proposed by the Quebec Task Force (1995) [71]

Grade	Presumed pathology	Clinical presentation
I	Microscopic or multimicroscopic lesion Lesion is not serious enough to cause muscle spasm	Usually presents to a doctor more than 24 h after trauma
II	Neck sprain and bleeding around soft tissue (articular capsules, ligaments, tendons, and muscles) Muscle spasm secondary to soft tissue injury	Usually presents to a doctor in the first 24 h after trauma Nonspecific radiation to the head, face, occipital region, shoulder, and arm form soft tissues injuries Neck pain with limited range of motion due to muscle spasm
III	Injuries to neurologic system by mechanical injury or by irritation secondary to bleeding or inflammation	Presents to a doctor usually within hours after the trauma Limited range of motion combined with neurologic symptoms and signs

Table 3. Summary of our classification

Degree	Lesion	Treatment
1st	Simple strain	Soft collar, 20 days
2nd	Strain	Soft collar with a good containment, 20 days
3rd	Serious strain	Hard collar, 25/30 days
4th	Compromising of mechanical stability	Minerva in Articast, 30/40 days
5th	Articular dislocation and or bony fractures	Surgery

in various studies. Nonetheless, it was surprising, and for us very pleasant, to discover the similarities.

To Immobilise or not to Immobilise: That Is the Question

We discuss this issue because our proposal is somewhat different from what can be found in the recent literature.

One of the biggest problems that we have to face nowadays regarding harmless spinal pathologies is if rest or early mobilisation is the best treatment. In some ways, low back pain and whiplash injury are similar because the general consensus of treatment by rest (should it be bed rest or collars) has shifted to a less general, but still common, consensus in promoting mobility as early as possible.

The Quebec Task Force on Whiplash Associated Disorders stated: "Based on limited evidence and reasoning by analogy, it is the Task Force consensus that the use of non steroid anti-inflammatory and analgesics, short-term manipulation and mobilisation by trained persons, and active exercises are useful in Grade II and III WAD, but prolonged use of soft collars, rest or inactivity probably prolongs disability in WAD".

In any case, this consensus does not mean that it is proven that mobilising is the correct answer to the problem, particularly in the case of a whiplash injured patient.

We have to remember that:
- All the studies addressing the problem have evaluated short term disability, but we know that long term results should be the most important for this type of patients.
- Soft collars do not immobilise the neck, but only restrict wide range movements.
- Mobilisation must be in any case a step in the treatment that we proposed, but this does not mean that must it be the first one.

- Many times the inadequate results of patients that have used a collar are due to the lack of a good rehabilitative process after removing the collar.
- Doctors must not abdicate their role of making the diagnosis and choosing treatments according to the level of pathology: research results say only what is better for most (statistical significance), not for all.

Bearing in mind these points, we think that it is not sound to propose, as many do, that mobilisation should be prescribed until it has been shown that immobilisation is superior to mobilising interventions.

Whiplash is presumably a form of distortion of the cervical spine. This pathogenic mechanism acts on a composed structure made up of many articulations, a large quantity of muscles with a very fine regulation and large bands with a stabilising, not a blocking function.

An orthopaedic general rule is that ligamentous or capsular stretchings require immobilisation as a means of repair. This must be prolonged to at least 18 days to be effective. Immobilisation can be partial or total according to the severity of pathology; it is also possible to prolong the immobilisation time according to necessity.

The real goal of treatment is to avoid over time pain and development of a possible instability at a distance. Our experience over the years has taught us that a cervical, whiplash injured spine that did not remained immobilised sufficiently can more frequently cause problems and that these problems last for a longer time.

Therefore, mobilisation is possible only if the trauma is so minor that there has not been a real lesion of ligamentous structures, but only a lengthening. If there is an involvement of capsules, ligaments or tendons, it will be necessary to immobilise.

We think that only when mobilisation proves more effective than immobilisation will it be possible not to observe these cautious rules.

Different Rehabilitative Tools

In this section we will compare our experience with the Quebec Task Force on Whiplash-Associated Disorders findings and our own search in the literature.

Physical Exercise

Physical exercise plays a major role in rehabilitating the patient integrating him back to a normal life. It is possible to identify some goals to be obtained: these can be achieved with very different techniques.

Pain Relief. Many exercise techniques able to reduce pain do exist and can be used in conjunction with decontracting and strengthening manoeuvres when one begins to remove the collar. We can mention, for example, the McKenzie method, the Mézières, Souchard or Bienfait approaches, the Sohier or Maitland technique and so on. Obviously The Method does not exist, but only many useful techniques that must fit the pathology of a single patient and the knowledge and ability of the physiotherapist.

Decontraction. This is usually the very first step. It can be achieved by relaxing the patient, letting him feel confident with the therapist. This is easier for example in a good environment, as happens in water, but for everybody it is suggested to work gradually, with the head well fixed at the beginning resting on the table, then in therapist's hands with a very good manual grasp.

This moment is not only muscular (and psychological) relaxation: it is also a first step in returning a part of the body to it's normal life. This means that exterofection and proprioception play a role other than the simple goal of decontraction.

Massage and infrared can help at this stage.

Strengthening. The evidence suggests that exercise may be beneficial in the short and long term. According to our experience, regaining enough strength to permit not only movement but usually also the ability to sustain the head is perhaps the most important goal when rehabilitation begins. The collar reduces the muscular usage, provoking deactivation that combines with injury and pain to reduce strength and trophism of muscular tissue.

This stage of rehabilitation constitutes also a very important step in regaining proprioceptive input from the muscular and articular tissues.

There are some techniques that are fundamental and cannot be ignored during this stage of treatment: isometric strengthening and rhythmic stabilisation. The first one constitutes a type of contraction more than a real technique and must be done at the beginning in a neutral position along the classical axes of movement, then at different degrees of movement as well as the intermediate plane. This is very important because the muscular tonic fibres are prevalent in the neck musculature due to it's physiological role, and because the first step is to permit to the head to be stable over it's "slender column".

The second technique involves movements effectuated by the patient with the opposition of the therapist provoking isometric and eccentric contractions along different axes of movement. This technique greatly increases both the strength and also the proprioceptive input.

Mobilisation. Having gained strength it is then necessary to gain mobility too. As we saw, it is possible to recover both together, but it is also wise to include in a good programme exercises along all the axes of movement, not ignoring the protraction/retraction movement. These exercises at the beginning will be passive and conducted by the therapist while respecting the pain. As both the patient and the therapist will become more confident pain will be explored more, particularly using active (assisted or not) contraction to avoid overstretching. Active exercises are very useful at this stage, and also automobilisation can be applied. The literature suggests that these techniques can be used as an adjunct to strategies that promote activation and that they can be beneficial particularly in the short term.

Normalisation. There are techniques developed to "normalise" the joint positions. These can be more or less gentle, depending on the method. They are an important way to regain good articular positioning, normalising in this way the afferents, reducing muscular hypercontraction, and avoiding pain. Studies about these techniques have not been published.

Proprioception. As has been sufficiently stressed above, proprioception plays a fundamental role in all the rehabilitation programmes, permitting good range of movements once it is possible. We do not think that neurology is the key to open the door of orthopaedic rehabilitation, as others involved in rehabilitation have proposed, but we are conscious of the importance of not neglecting this fundamental element.
    This goal of the treatment is not discussed in the literature.

Posture. The literature does not address this item as a single therapeutic element; rather, many researchers have proposed it as a part of a multimodal treatment plan.
    We think that it is not possible to only propose a local intervention, because the neck has a function: let the eyes look forward. This function must be accomplished independently by the various elements, and this means based on the posture of the rest of the body. This posture must be compensated by the neck. This is why it is of enormous importance to intervene and modify the posture of the body if we want to prevent other stresses on the neck.

Activity of Daily Life. The neck must be used 24 h per day, 7 days per week, 52 weeks per year. Any activity could be more or less stressful for this already lesioned structure. How to sit, how to work, how to sleep are not only insignificant to the rehabilitation programme.
    In this case, as in the next one, lack of literature does not mean lack of sense.

Thoracic and Lumbar Spine. Finally, when rehabilitating a neck it is not possible to neglect the other parts of the spine. The vertebral column in fact has been defined as one, articulated long bone, and an injury in one part always reflects on the other (apart from a lesion developed during the injury itself). This is why it is very important to consider the thoracic and lumbar regions too.

Active Participation of the Patient. Therapists used to think that a patient must rely on them and that without their help the patient will not be able to work properly. Perhaps this is true, but what is much more important is what the patient loses by not working on his own. Working at home is fundamental, and particularly isometric exercises and the ones necessary to regain mobility can be done and controlled without many problems. This is a must.

This goal is well known in the literature, but specific studies about this topic do not exist.

Physical Therapy

The main goal of physical therapy is to promote soft tissue healing and to diminish inflammation. A part from magnetotherapy, studies addressing exclusively this issue do not exist.

Magnetotherapy. There are results in the literature about the association between use of a collar and continued magnetotherapy with benefits in the short term. In our experience, it is possible to prescribe a 20 min application for at least 20 times: usually it is necessary to use 60 Gauss with a frequency of five times a week.

Laser Therapy. It can be useful if trigger points can be detected. Particularly useful, in our experience, are the He-Ne and the As-Ga lasers.

Heat. Many time heat has to be proscribed in the cervical region, and this is particularly true in whiplash injury: the sympathetic plexus is placed around the vertebral artery and can be influenced by this type of treatment with dangerous effect, particularly when a lesion is suspected here. Vertigo can commonly appear using heat in the cervical region, and that is why, when vertigo is a major complaint, it is better not to try this type of therapy.

Infrared is very superficial and could be used, with some cautions, associated with massage.

Radar therapy and Marconi rays are forbidden because of the heat that develops, as is the case for ultrasound therapy, which could micromassage the soft tissues.

Electrotherapy. This type of therapy is not so useful. TENS can reduce pain, iontophoresis can have an anti-inflammatory effect, but their importance is not very great in whiplash injured patients.

Cold. This type of therapy does not have a great significance and is not usually used in such cases.

Mechanical Therapy

The most important danger in treating whiplash is excessive mobilisation of a structure not completely repaired. This is what could happen with all manual therapies, and this is why it is necessary to be very cautious, particularly if the healing process could not be completed.

Manipulation. This is a common treatment but its value has not been established till now.

According to our experience it is inappropriate in whiplashed patients, because it is possible to obtain mobility and a pain free situation with less risks using simple exercises.

Massage. Massage can be applied, but it must be relaxing to reduce muscular contraction particularly just before and after physical exercise therapy.

Traction. There is only one study addressing the problem of traction of pathological necks, but it did not focus on whiplash and its results were not definitive.

The most important danger with this treatment is the damage to soft tissues, with overstretching of ligaments, capsule of zygapophyseal joints and (less important) muscles. This is always present to a lesser or greater degree, and this is why traction, according to our thought, must not be applied.

References

1. Algers G, Pettersson K, Hildingsson C, Toolanen G (1993) Surgery for chronic symptoms after whiplash injury. Follow up of 20 cases. Acta Orthop Scand 64(6):654-656
2. Allen ME, Weir Jones I, Motiuk DR Flewin KR Goring RD, Kobetitch R Broadhurst A (1994) Acceleration perturbations of daily living. A comparison to "whiplash". Spine 19(11):1285-1290
3. Alpini D, Cesarani A, Sibilla P (1990) Dal piede alla corteccia. Il controllo extra-labirintico del sistema vestibolare. In: Dufour A (ed). 10 anni di ENG. Formenti Ed
4. Barnsley L, Lord S, Bogduk N (1993) Comparative local anaesthetic blocks in

the diagnosis of cervical zygapophysial joint pain. Pain 55(1):99-106

5. Barnsley L, Lord S, Bogduk N (1994) Whiplash injury. Pain 58(3): 283-307
6. Barnsley L, Lord SM, Wallis BJ, Bogduk N (1994) Lack of effect of intra-articular corticosteroids for chronic pain in the cervical zygapophyseal joints. N Engl J Med 330(15):1047-1050
7. Barry M (1992) Whiplash injuries. Br J Rheumatol 31(9):579-581
8. Bovim G, Schrader H, Sand T (1994) Neck pain in the general population. Spine 19(12):1307-1309
9. Bowen J, Patz J, Bailey J, Hansen K (1992) Dissection of vertebral artery after cervical trauma. Lancet 339(8790):435-436
10. Brodin H (1984) Cervical Pain and Mobilisation. Int J Rehabil Res 7:190-191
11. Byrn C, Olsson I, Falkheden L, Lindh M, Hosterey U, Fogelberg M, Linder LE, Bunketorp O (1993) Subcutaneous sterile water injections for chronic neck and shoulder pain following whiplash injuries. Lancet 341(8843):449-452
12. Carette S (1994) Whiplash injury and chronic neck pain. N Engl J Med, Apr 14, 330(15):1083-1084
13. Cassidy JD, Lopes AA, Yong-Hing K (1992) The immediate effect of manipulation on pain and range of motion in the cervical spine: a randomized controlle trial. J Manipulative Physiol Ther 15:570-575
14. Chester JB Jr (1991) Whiplash, postural control, and the inner ear. Spine 16(7):716-720
15. Colachis SC, Strohm BR, Ganter EL (1973) Cervical spine motion in normal women: radiographic study on effect of cervical collars. Arch Phys Med Rehabil 54:161-169
16. Da Cunha HM, Cesarani A, Ciancaglini R, Lazzari E, Ruyu A, Sibilla P (1994) Postura, Occlusione, Rachide. Edizioni CPA, Milano
17. Davis SJ, Teresi LM, Bradley WG Jr, Ziemba MA, Bloze AE (1991) Cervical spine hyperextension injuries: MR findings. Radiology 180(1):245-251
18. Dvorak J, Herdmann J, Janssen B, Theiler R, Grob D (1990) Motor evoked potentials in patients with cervical spine disorders. Spine 15(10):1013-1013
19. Dvorak J, Panjabi MM, Grob D, Novotny JE, Antinnes JA (1993) Clinical validation of functional flexion/extension radiographs of the cervical spine. Spine 18(1):120-127
20. Fischer AA (1993) Sterile water for whiplash syndrome. Lancet 341(8843):470
21. Fisher SV, Bowar JF, Awad EA, Gullikson G (1977) Cervical orthoses effect on cervical spine motion: roengenographic and goniometric method of study. Arch Phys Med Rehabil 58:109-115
22. Foley Nolan D, Barry C, Coughlan R, O'Comnor P (1990) Pulsed high frequency (27 Mhz) electromagnetic therapy for persistent neck pain. A double blind placebo controlled study of 20 patients. Orthopedics 13:445-451
23. Foley Nolan D, Moore K, Codd M, Barry C, O'Connor P, Coughlan RJ (1992) Low energy high frequency pulsed electromagnetic therapy for acute whiplash injuries. A double blind randomized controlled study. Scand J Rehabil Med 24(1):51-59
24. Galasko CS, Murray PM, Pitcher M, Chambers H, Mansfield S, Madden M, Jordon C, Kinsella A, Hodson M (1993) Neck sprains after road traffic accidents: a modern epidemic. Injury 24(3):155-157

25. Gargan M, Bannister G (1991) Soft tissue injuries to the neck. BMJ 303(6805):786

26. Gargan MF, Bannister GC (1990) Long term prognosis of soft tissue injuries of the neck. J Bone Joint Surg Br 72(5):901-903

27. Gebhard JS, Donaldson DH, Brown CW (1994) Soft tissue injuries the cervical spine. Orthop Rev, May, S:9-17

28. Hamer AJ, Gargan MF, Bannister GC, Nelson RJ (1993) Whiplash injury and surgically treated cervical disc disease. Injury 24(8):549-550

29. Harris JH, Yeakley JW (1992) Hyperextension dislocation of the cervical spine. Ligament injuries demonstrated by magnetic resonance imaging. J Bone Joint Surg Br 74(4):567-570

30. Hodgson SP, Grundy M (1989) Neck sprains after car accidents. BMJ 298(6685):1452

31. Horne G (1989) Neck sprains after car accidents. BMJ 299(6690):53

32. Johnson RM, Hart DL, Simmons EF, Ramsby GR, Southwick WO (1977) Cervical orthoses. A study comparing their effectiveness in restricting cervical motion in normal subjects. J Bone Joint Surg Am 59:332-339

33. Luo ZP, Goldsmith W (1991) Reaction of a human head/neck/torso system to shock. J Biomech 24(7):499-510

34. Magnusson T (1994) Extracervical symptoms after whiplash trauma. Cephalalgia 14(3):223-227

35. Maimaris C (1989) Neck sprains after car accidents. BMJ 299(6691):123

36. McKinney LA (1989) Early mobilisation and outcome in acute sprains of the neck. BMJ 299:1006-1008

37. McKinney LA, Dornan JO, Ryan M (1989) The role of physiotherapy in the management of acute neck sprains following road traffic accidents. Arch Emerg Med 6(1):27-33

38. Mealy K, Brennan H, Fenelon GC (1986) Early mobilisation of acute whiplash injuries. BMJ 292:656-657

39. Negrini A, Negrini S (1989) Il trattamento chinesiologico delle algie vertebrali. Chinesiologia Scientifica 3:51-57

40. Negrini A, Negrini S (1994) La cinesiterapia secondo Charrière. In: Negrini S (ed). La cinesiterapia nel trattamento delle lombalgie: metodi a confronto. Vigevano, Gruppo di Studio della Scoliosi delle patologie vertebrali, 51-61

41. Negrini A jr, Negrini S, Santambrogio GC (1994) Data variability in the analysis of spinal deformity: a study performed by means of the Auscan System. In: D'Amico M, Merolli A, Santambrogio GC (eds). Three-dimensional analysis of spinal deformities. Amsterdam, IOS, 101-106

42. Negrini S, Negrini A jr, Rainero G, Sibilla P, Santambrogio GC (1994) Correlation between trunk gibbosity and the spinal torsion measured by the Auscan System. In: D'Amico M, Merolli A, Santambrogio GC (eds). Three-dimensional analysis of spinal deformities. Amsterdam, IOS, 279-283

43. Negrini S, Negrini A jr, Santambrogio GC, Sibilla P (1994) Relation between static angles of the spine and a dynamic eventi like posture: approach to the problem. In: D'Amico M, Merolli A, Santambrogio GC (eds). Three dimensional analysis of spinal deformities. Amsterdam, IOS, 209-214

44. Negrini S, Negrini A jr (1992) Algie vertebrali croniche e disturbi dell'equilibrio:

risultati preliminari dell'esame con "Balance Platform". La Ginnastica Medica 40(1/2/3):29-35

45. Negrini S (1994) La cinesiterapia nel trattamento delle lombalgie: metodi a confronto. Vigevano, Gruppo di Studio della Scoliosi e delle patologie vertebrali

46. Negrini S (1994) Metodologia nella cinesiterapia per il paziente lombalgico. In: Negrini S (ed). La cinesiterapia nel trattamento delle lombalgie: metodi a confronto. Vigevano, Gruppo di Studio della Scoliosi e delle patologie vertebrali, 3-21

47. Negrini S (1994) La terapia meccanica di McKenzie. In: Negrini S (ed). La cinesiterapia nel trattamento delle lombalgie: metodi a confronto. Vigevano, Gruppo di Studio della Scoliosi e delle patologie vertebrali, 83-97

48. Newman PK (1990) Whiplash injury. BMJ 301(6749):395-396

49. Pearce JM (1989) Whiplash injury: a reappraisal. J Neurol Neurosurg Psychiatry 52(12):1329-1331

50. Pearce JM (1990) Whiplash injury. BMJ 301(6752):610

51. Pearce JM (1993) Pain relief by water injections. Lancet 341(8849):905

52. Pearce JM (1993) Subtle cerebral lesions in "chronic whiplash syndrome"? J Neurol Neurosurg Psychiatry 56(12):1328-1329

53. Pearce JM (1993) Polemics of chronic whiplash injury. Neurology 44(11):1993-1997

54. Pennie B, Agambar L (1991) Patterns of injury and recovery in whiplash. Injury 22(1):57-59

55. Pennie BH, Agambar LJ (1990) Whiplash injuries. A trial of early management. J Bone Joint Surg Br 72(2):277-279

56. Pettersson K, Hildingsson C, Toolanen G, Fagerlund M, Bjornebrink J (1994) MRI and neurology in acute whiplash trauma. No correlation in prospective examination of 39 cases. Acta Orthop Scand 65(5):525-528

57. Porter KM (1989) Neck sprains after car accidents. BMJ 298(6679):973-974

58. Radanov BP, Di Stefano G, Schnidrig A, Sturzenegger M (1994) Common whiplash: psychosomatic or somatopsychic'? J Neurol Neurosurg Psychiatry 57(4):486-490

59. Radanov BP, Di Stefano G, Schnidrig A, Sturzenegger M, Augustiny KF (1993) Cognitive functioning after common whiplash. A controlled follow-up study. Arch Neurol 50(1):87-91

60. Radanov BP, Dvorak J, Valach L (1992) Cognitive deficits in patients after soft tissue injury of the cervical spine. Spine 17(2):127-131

61. Radanov BP, Schnidrig A, Di Stefano G, Sturzenegger M (1992) Illness behaviour after common whiplash. Lancet 339(8795):749-750

62. Radanov BP, Sturzenegger M, De Stefano G, Schnidrig A (1994) Relationship between early somatic, radiological. cognitive and psychosocial findings and outcome during a one year follow up in 117 patients suffering from common whiplash. Br J Rheumatol 33(5):442-448

63. Redmond AD (1992) Prognostic factors in soft tissue injuries of the cervical spine. Injury 23(4):285

64. Shea M, Wittenberg RH, Edwards WT, White AA 3d, Hayes WC (1992) In vitro hyperextension injuries in the human cadaveric cervical spine. J Orthop Res 10(6):911-916

65. Sibilla P (1990) Scoliosi, modello d'interazione spino-vertebrale. In: Cesarani

186

A, Alpini D (eds). Diagnosi e trattamento dei disturbi dell'equilibrio. Mediamix, Milano, 19-28

66. Sibilla P, Cesarani A, Barozzi S, Alpini D, Rainero G (1990) Scoliosis: a model to evaluate spino-vestibular interactions. In: Claussen CF (ed). NES Congress Proceedings, Bad Kissingen

67. Sibilla P, Cesarani A, Barozzi S, Alpini D, Rainero G (1991) Scoliosis: a model to evaluate spino-vestibular interactions". In: Claussen CF (ed). Vertigo, nausea, tinnitus and hypoacusia due to head and neck trauma. Elsevier Science, 225-228

68. Sibilla P, Cesarani A, Negrini S. Atanasio S, Alpini D, Romano M, Barozzi S (1994) Stepping coordination in scoliosis evaluated by the mean of craniocorpography. In: Taguchi K, Igarashi M, Mori S (eds). Vestibular and neural front. Amsterdam, Elsevier Science BV, 39-42

69. Sibilla P, Atanasio S, Fronte F, Santambrogio GC (1994) Three dimensional evaluation of scoliosis progression during pregnancy: a non ionising study. In: D'Amico M, Merolli A, Santambrogio GC (eds). Three dimensional analysis of spinal deformities. Amsterdam, IOS, 293-296

70. Simons DG (1989) Myofascial trigger points and the whiplash syndrome. Clin J Pain 5(3):279

71. Spitzer WO, Skovron ML, Salmi LR, Cassidy JD, Duranceau J, Suissa S, Zeiss E (1995) Scientific Monograph of the Quebec Task Force on Whiplash-Associated Disorders. Redefining "Whiplash" and its management. Spine (8S):20

72. Sturzenegger M, Di Stefano G, Radanov BP, Schnidrig A (1994) Presenting symptoms and signs after whiplash injury: the influence of accident mechanisms. Neurology 44(4):688-693

73. Taylor JR, Kakulas BA (1991) Neck injuries. Lancet 338(8778):1343

74. Watkinson AF (1990) Whiplash injury. BMJ 301(6758):983

75. Watkinson A, Gargan MF, Bannister GC (1991) Prognostic factors in soft tissue injuries of the cervical spine. Injury 22(4):307-309

76. Winters JM, Peles JD, Osterbauer PJ, Derickson K, Deboer KF. Fuhr AW (1993) Three-dimensional head axis of rotation during tracking movements. A tool for assessing neck neuromechanical function. Spine 18(9):1178-1185

77. Woltring HJ, Long K, Osterbauer PJ, Fuhr AW (1994) Instantaneous helical axis estimation from 3D video data in neck kinematics for whiplash diagnostics. J Biomech 27(12):1415-1432

78. Zylbergold RS, Piper MC (1985) Cervical spine disorders. A comparison of three types of traction. Spine 10:867-871

79. Whiplash injury. Lancet 338(8776):1207-1208

Acupuncture and Neuroreflexology

P. L. Ghilardi, C. Borsari[1], A. Casani, L. Bonuccelli and B. Fattori

Introduction

Acupuncture [26] may be considered a valid and efficacious tool in the treatment of cervically originated vertigo since it intervenes on a known physiopathological substrate [7]. It exerts its function through the activation of the transducers in the skin and in the surface and deep muscles in the neck, which are capable of affecting the vestibulo-spinal reflex arc [5, 27]. It is well known, in fact, that vestibulo-spinal reflexes play a fundamentally important role in the maintenance of posture [1]. Experiments on animals have shown that the neurons of the lateral reticular nucleus (LRN), the bulbar relay station of the ascending somatosensorial pathway, are responsive to lateral tilting [15]. The response of these LRN neurons to head tilting does not appear to depend on either peripheral proprioception or skin feedback. While the LRN can receive signals from the macular receptors directly through Deiter's lateral vestibular nucleus (LVN), responses to tilting can be also mediated, to a certain extent, by an indirect influence of the lateral vestibulo-spinal tract on the ascending neurons of the reticulo-spinal pathway [4]. It has already been demonstrated that the lateral vestibulo-spinal tract stimulates the extensor motoneurons of the lower limb muscles in a monosynaptic manner, whereas the descending fibers in the ventral quadrant, including those in the lateral vestibulo-spinal tract, are capable of exerting a monosynaptic stimulus in the neurons with ascending axons in the ventrolateral cord. These ascending neurons have bilateral receptive fields and respond to the stimulation of high threshold cutaneous and muscle fiber afferents (flexion reflex afferents, FRA) which often originate in the four limbs [8]. It is believed that this ascending tract, called the bilateral ventral flexion reflex tract, or bVFRT, projects towards neurons which are situated both in the main reticular formation and in the LRN [8]. This pathway seems to be organised in a rather diffusive manner as compared with the peripheral somatic input transmission and could well have an important function in the head and body

Institute of Otorhinolaryngology, University of Pisa, Pisa, Italy
[1] 3rd Department of Anesthesiology, St. Chiara Hospital, Pisa, Italy

for distinguishing orientation, particularly with respect to a possible influence descending from the vestibular structures. The rostral-ventral and caudal-dorsal parts of the LVN, which project towards the cervical and sacro-lumbar segments of spinal cord respectively, are known to be influenced in a differential manner by the labyrinthine and cervical afferents. A response pattern opposite to that of the individual macular and cervical inputs has been seen in the Purkinje cells of the cerebellar vermis which projects towards the LVN, indicating that cerebellar elaboration can take part in the production of opposing patterns in the discharge frequency of the LVN neurons for the same direction of movement or of rotation of the neck [16]. The stimuli issued by the macular and labyrinthine receptors and transmitted to the descending vestibulo-spinal system are well-known to be involved in the maintenance of posture [10, 21]. When the head or neck is bent or when the head alone is turned after elimination of the cervical reflexes, there are pronounced changes in the discharge activity of the LVN neurons and particularly in the population of neurons which transmit to the cervico-spinal segments through the lateral vestibulo-spinal pathway. This finding is in agreement with the fact that, from an anatomical point of view, the lateral vestibulo-spinal pathway which originates in the LVN has a somatotopical-like organisation and the primary vestibular afferents associated with the macular receptors terminate prevalently in the rostro-ventral portion of this nucleus, the neurons of which transmit to the cervical segments of the spinal cord [23]. The relative effects of tilting on the muscles in the neck and in the upper and lower limbs and on the spinal motoneurons indicate that the tonic motor responses evoked by the labyrinth tend to contrast with tilting and to bring the head and trunk back to their normal stance [24, 25]. In view of the above-mentioned physiopathological considerations, we believe that acupuncture stimulation acts by activating the reflexes originating in the skin and muscles (FRA) which transmit, through the bVFRT to the latero-reticular nucleus neurons in the brainstem [8]. Neurophysiological experiments have demonstrated how stimuli starting in the nape muscles can not only modulate the discharge activity of the neurons in the latero-reticular nucleus but can also modify the frequency of the discharge of vermis cortex neurons in the anterior cerebellar lobe through activation of the ascending cerebellar reticulo-spinal pathway [9, 4]. The Purkinje cells in this part of the cerebellar cortex transmit important signals down to Deiters LVN [15] which is one of the principal structures in the vestibulo-spinal reflex arc. Posture is a complex nervous function which has been studied throughout time with various dated clinical methods, the most classical example of which is without doubt Romberg's manoeuvre. Nowadays it is possible to study postural function with computerised methods, which permit very objective evaluations in almost real time, by means of stabilometric systems. With this method it is possible to assess the integrity of the spinal vestibular reflex (SVR) which contributes to antigravitational muscular activity [20]. The duty of postural function is to keep a body upright, against the dynamical threats exerted by gravity and by voluntary and involuntary movement of the head and body, but it also has the task of stabilising the visual field according to the head's movement. Stabilometric systems permit studying the upright position by recording the reflex activity which is the basis of this position; in other words, balance is a dynamic condition since there has to be a series of permanent muscle reactions which must adequately compensate the continuous variations in the centre of gravity as the body moves. Stabilometry not only records the position with reference to the centre of gravity on the ground but it also reveals dynamic effects linked to the accelerations due to activity of the muscles which have the task of avoiding falls (inverted pendulum model) as shifts in the centre of pressure occur. This is to say that the stabilometric tracing interprets as further shifts in gravity even these dynamic effects, which actually have an opposite motor effect [12].

Our Clinical Experience

The above mentioned physiopathological considerations prompted us to apply acupuncture (particularly as reflex therapy) to disorders in which there is a prevalent alteration in the macular and cervical inputs; this is seen at its utmost in trauma from cervical torsion. In fact, in these patients particularly there is an alteration in the cervical proprioceptive inputs due to stretching of the neuromuscular spindles and the osteo-tendon articulation receptors in the neck [14]. In patients affected by balance disorders of cervical origin and particularly in those with whiplash injury (WI) there is a prevalence of postural disorders linked with alterations in the VSR (vestibulo-spinal reflex) over those related to VOR (vestibulo-ocular reflex). For this reason, posturographic examination appears to be the most appropriate method for both qualitative and quantitative clinical assessment of the alterations in the postural patterns of these patients and for monitoring their follow up [17, 19]. Posturographic examination is performed first of all in OE conditions (open eyes) with the patients gazing at an illuminated spot, then in CE (closed eyes). In this routine posture test we also used sensitisation tests to eliminate and/or disturb one or two of the three sensitive entrances to the posture system (visual, proprio-exteroceptive and vestibular). Two of these tests which we routinely applied were the head retroflexion test (CER) and the head shaking posturographic test (CE HST). The posturographic examination of the patient was performed, during the first session, with three investigations consisting each of four tests: OE; CE; CER; CEHST. The first investigation was performed in basal conditions. The second was carried out after simulating acupuncture; that is, by placing four needles on random points of the cervical region so that the patient could feel only subjective stimulation. This simulation of acupuncture before the true acupuncture session served to exclude the presence of functional components. The third investigation was performed immediately after the actual acupuncture. Thereafter, further sessions were carried out once a week for 3-5 weeks according to the patient's clinical response and they were always monitored with posturography. Acupuncture was performed by piercing deeply and bilaterally points 10V (Tienn Chou) and 20VB (Fong Tcheou) with steel needles which were twirled manually for 20 s after insertion. Each session lasted 20 min. We chose these acupuncture points on the basis of the long established Chinese experience in this field [3, 28] and also on our own previous studies [3]. However, other points may be used with equal results (17TR, 3IG, 62V, ear points, scalp puncture, etc.) though we have not used them in order to maintain uniformity in the investigation. The posturographic examination in our patients with WI confirmed alterations in both OE and CE in 45% of the cases, though no specific pattern could be distinguished. The stabilogram gave a prevalence of wide and arrythmic oscillations on both planes, though the sagittal plane prevailed over the other (Fig. 1). The statokinetic parametres showed an increase, particularly in the surface. The centre of gravity often appeared shifted to one side (Fig. 2).

These findings were seen to be altered even more in the sensitisation tests, particularly when the head was retroflexed (Fig. 3). In CE and CER, analysis

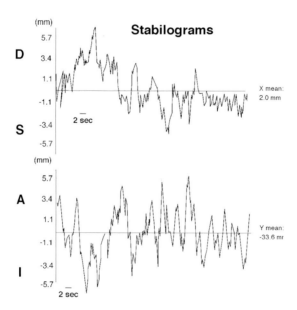

Fig. 1. Stabilograms: prevalence of wide and arythmic oscillations on both planes, with prevalence on sagittal plane

Statokinesigram

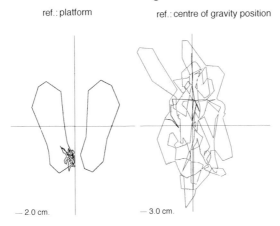

ref.: platform   ref.: centre of gravity position

— 2.0 cm.   — 3.0 cm.

Fig. 2. Statokinesigram: the centre of gravity appears shifted to the left

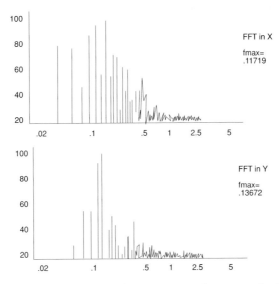

Fig. 3. Test performed in CE: the Fourier spectrogram shows a maximal frequency peak on 0.1-0.2 Hz

of the Fourier spectrogram revealed frequencies shifted towards 0.1-0.2 Hz (Fig. 4). After the first acupuncture session in our experiment we noticed an improvement in stance in 75% of our patients. Nevertheless, this resulted was transient in the majority of cases; once the acupuncture sessions were repeated this improvement tended to stabilise. After the three to five ses-

Statokinesigram

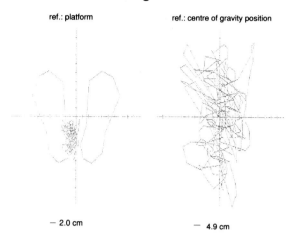

ref.: platform   ref.: centre of gravity position

— 2.0 cm   — 4.9 cm

Fig. 4. CER test: the statokinesigram shows a remarkable increase of surface

sions of acupuncture on our group of patients with cervical torsion trauma, 60%-70% of the balance disorders were cured, whereas 20% showed considerable improvement as compared with the initial conditions. The results were nonsatisfactory in only 10%-20% of the patients, either because of a lack of response to acupuncture treatment or due to rapid regression of the improvement achieved once the sessions were over. Cervical torsion trauma, and balance disorders with cervical origin in general, such as those connected with pronounced antalgic contracture of the nape muscles due to cervical arthrosis, are the conditions which responded best to acupuncture. In fact, other groups of patients suffering from vertigo of other natures did not respond so well.

In central type disorders (vasculopathies or neurodegeneration) we saw no positive response to acupuncture in any of the patients we treated and who were always submitted to posturography in the same manner as described before. In the cases of monolateral peripheral vestibular deficiency we encountered positive reponses to acupuncture in 35%, while no statistically significant improvement ($p > 0.1$) was seen in the posturography performed in the group of patients with cupulolithiasis [18, 11].

Conclusions

Posture study with the aid of a stabilometric platform can supply an objective assessment of acupuncture efficacy, particularly in patients with balance disorders of cervical origin. In fact, the stabilometric examination permits quantifying the various postural parametres and gives a graphic description of any shifting in pressure centres on both sagittal and transversal planes, hence it is possible to perform a series of repeated tests which are perfectly comparable with each other. The patients suffering from central type vertigo disorders, mainly vascular, showed very few variations in stance both before and after acupuncture. The most interesting results were accomplished in the group of patients with balance disorders of cervical origin; these cases showed satisfactory results right from the first acupuncture session and the postural parametres of the four stabilometric tests became normal in 75% of the cases. Even the patients with peripheral vestibular disorders, particularly monolateral vestibular damage, had interesting results with an improvement in posture performance in 35% of the cases, which can very likely be attributed to a plastic and self corrective rebuilding of the VSR arc produced by acupuncture. Acupuncture stimulation in these situations appears to activate the ascending reticulo-spinal cerebellar pathways and, therefore, the descending projections which, from the cortical vermis area of the anterior lobe of the cerebellum, modulate the activity of the Deiters LVN, the basis of the VSR. There are many clinical reports which confirm the efficacy of acupuncture in balance disorders when performed according to the traditional methods established by ancient Chinese energetic medicine, but there are very few experimental data referring to the neurophysiological and/or neuroendocrinological mechanisms of action of acupuncture in vertigo of cervical origin. In recent years much progress has been accomplished regarding the anatomy and physiology of the acupuncture points but, above all, modern acupuncture specialists have shifted their interest towards research into the physiological aspects of the points. Present-day research is still far from a thorough explanation of acupuncture and many hypotheses have been pronounced on this matter: the mechanisms of action are quite definitely many [22]. Acupuncture is certainly capable of interfering with the mechanism of action of numerous neurotransmitters (endogenous oppoids, serotonin, P substance, catecholamine, GABA, cortisol, etc.) [6] and it also provokes excitation reflexes and inhibition of the spinal cord (grey gel substance of the periaqueduct), of the bulbar areas (reticular substance) and of the thalamic and cortical regions [2, 13]. Another possible mechanism of action which must be considered, especially in cases of vertigo of cervical origin, is a sympathicolytic action exerted via inhibition of the brainstem reticular substance. These data indicate that this treatment is capable of directly modifying the reflexes which start from the cervical region and and which are responsible for balance disorders. One must also take into account an antiedema activity, however, which can reduce the effects of pressure on the posterior roots of the cervical nerves, and also a more generalised activity of stabilisation of the basilar vertebral system. The positive effects became manifest immediately after even just one acupuncture session; nevertheless, in this experiment we noticed a decrease in efficacy during the following days which required a series of further sessions of acupuncture in order to stabilise the results, as seen in the follow-up of these patients. The high percentage of positive responses, particularly in the cases of vertigo of cervical origin and less so in those with monolateral peripheral vestibular deficiency, leads us to advocate the therapeutic efficacy of acupuncture, at least in disorders in which it can be associated with or proven as a valid alternative to pharmacological treatment.

References

1. Abrahams VC, Richmond FJR (1988) Specialization of sensorimotor organization in the neck muscle system. In: Pompeiano O, Allum JHJ (eds). Vestibulospinal control of posture and locomotion. Progress in Brain Research, Elsevier, 76:125-135
2. Baohian P, Li G (1993) The ultrastructure and enzyme histocheminstry of the substantia gelatinosa of rat spinal cord under the influence of electroacupuncture analgesie. World J Acup Mox 3:43-48
3. Bonuccelli L, Fattori B, Ghilardi PL, Casani A, Vatteroni UR, Capetta M (1991) Agopuntura e vertigine cervicale: valutazione posturografica. Giornale Italiano di Riflessologia e Agopuntura 3:2-3
4. Boyle R, Pompeiano O (1981) Convergence and Interaction of Neck and Macular Vestibular Inputs on Vestibulospinal neurons. J Neurophysiol 45:852-868
5. Chan SHH, Fung SF (1975) Suppression of polysynaptic reflex by electro-acupuncture and a possible underlying mechanism in the spinal cord of the cat. Exp Neurol 48:336-342
6. Chen Zheng Qiu (1993) Partecipation of GABA in SII emanating descending modulation on the nucleus centrum medianum in motor cortex in acupuncture analgesia. Word Journal of Acupuncture and Moxibustion 3:46-50
7. Coan RM, Wong G, Coan PL (1982) The acupuncture treatment of neck pain: a randomized controlled study. Am J Clin Med 9:327-332
8. Coulter JD, Mergner T, Pompeiano O (1975) Effects of static tilt on cervical spinoreticular tract neurons. J Neurophysiol 39:45-62
9. Denoth F, Magherini PC, Pompeiano O, Stanojevic M (1980) Responses of Purkinje cells of cerebellar vermis to sinusoidal rotation of neck. J Neurophysiol 43:46-59
10. Fujita Y, Rosenberg J, Segundo JP (1968) Activity of cells in the lateral vestibular nucleus as a function of head position. J Physiol 196:1-18
11. Ghilardi PL, Fattori B, Casani A, Piragine F (1990) La posturografia nei deficit unilaterali vestibolari periferici. Acta Otorhinol Ital 10:347-356
12. Gurfinkel EV (1973) Physical foundation of stabilography. Agressologie 14C:9-14
13. Han J (1988) Central neurotransmitters and acupuncture analgesia In: Pomeranz B, Stux G (eds). Scientific bases of acupuncture. Springer, Berlin, Heidelberg, New York, pp 7-33

14. Hinoki M, Niki H (1975) Neurogical studies on the role of the sympathetic nervous system in the information of traumatic vertigo of cervical origin. Acta Otolaryngol, Stockh [Suppl 330]:185-196
15. Kubin L, Manzoni D, Pompeiano O (1981) Responses of lateral reticular neurons to convergent neck and macular vestibular inputs. J Neurophysiol 46:48-64
16. Lindsay KW, Roberts TDM Rosemberg JR (1976) Asymmetric tonic labyrinth reflexes and their interaction with neck reflexes in the decerebrated cats. J Physiol, London, 261:583-601
17. Norré ME, Forrez G (1985a) Application otoneurologiques cliniques de la posturographie. Les Cahiers d'ORL 20:255-273
18. Norré ME, Forrez G (1985b) La posturographie dans la pathologie vestibulaire périphérique. Ann Oto-Laryngol 102:503-509
19. Norré ME, Forrez G, Stevens A, Beckers A (1987) Cervical vertigo diagnosed by posturography? Preliminary report. Acta ORL Belgica 41:574-581
20. Norré ME, Forrez G, Beckers A (1988) Posturographie et rééducation vestibulaire. Les Cahiers d'ORL 23:11-19
21. Peterson BV (1970) Distribution of neural responses to tilting within vestibular nuclei of the cat. J Neurophysiol 33:750-767
22. Pomeranz B, Stux G (1988) Scientific bases of acupuncture. Springer, Berlin, Heidelberg, New York
23. Pompeiano O, Brodal A (1957) The origin of vestibulospinal fibers in the cat. An experimental-anatomical study, with comments on the descending medial longitudinal fasciculus. Arch Ital Biol 95:166-195
24. Roberts TDM (1973) Reflex balance. Nature 244:156-158
25. Rosenberg JR, Lindsay KW (1973) Asymmetric tonic labyrinthine reflexes. Brain Res 63:347-350
26. Senelar R (1979) Les caractéristiques morphologiques des points chinois. In: Niboyet GEH (ed). Nouveau Traité d'Acupuncture. Maisonneuve, pp 249-277
27. Zhang S, Luo Y, Bo M (1991) Vertigo treatment with scalp acupuncture. J Tradit Chin Medicine 11:26-28
28. Zizzo A, Ercolani M (1990) La vertigine. AMAB, IV Congresso di Agopuntura, La Neurologia, pp 29-34

Physiotherapy of the Neck, Back and Pelvis in Patients with Whiplash Injuries

I. ÖDKVIST AND L. ÖDKVIST[1]

Introduction

Whiplash injuries entail lesions in the cervical spine. There may be elongations of ligaments, smaller or more serious vertebral fractures, disc compressions, proplapses or dislocations of vertebrae.

The treatment strategy depends upon the type and degree of cervical lesion. Stabilising surgery may be indicated in severe cases. Psychological approaches are a necessity. Simultaneous damage to the brain, brainstem, inner ear, back, pevis or lower extremities has to be taken into consideration when planning treatment. Physiotherapy in whiplash injuries has a central role.

Assessment of Damage

In order to assess the lesions, case history, clinical investigation, and imaging with radiology and MRI are mandatory. This should be performed before the patient is seen by the physiotherapist.

The manual examination sometimes has to be postponed due to the cervical pain. The degree of active movement is of importance to notice. Pain may contraindicate some parts of the examination and physiotherapy, especially in the acute stage.

Neck hyperextension and dislocation should be noticed and may contraindicate most physiotherapeutic manouvres. One must proceed with caution in implementing neck therapy if the assessment is not performed in an adequate way by the responsible physician and in some parts completed by the physiotherapist. Cervical lesions may be worsened by too brisk examinations.

Physiotherapy, Risbrinksgatan 6a, Linköping, Sweden
[1] Department of Otolaryngology, University Hospital, Linköping, Sweden

Treatment

In the *acute stage* painkillers and anti-inflammatory drugs such as NSAIDs may be given. The physiotherapist, in the first 24 h, can use cold packs to prevent pain, unnecessary tissue swelling and oedema. A soft, supporting cervical collar should be used the first few days after injury. The collar offers support for the neck and head in a pain-free position with the neck in a favourable position. After a few days the collar should be taken off a number of times each day. During these hours the neck is trained with gradually increasing active exercises. It is important to know that the recovery is not delayed by not using the collar. Short periods of collar use are suggested by some authors [1]. The patient should avoid excessive use of the collar, which could cause bad posture and delay mobilisation [2]. The collar may also be suitable for nocturnal use. The patient should avoid sleeping on the stomach as this causes an extreme extension and sometimes rotation of the cervical spine.

For sleeping a suitable pillow is advisable, offering support to the head with the head in a median position and the cervical muscles relaxed.

In the acute phase acupuncture has its role for pain relief starting carefully as soon as possible after the accident and increasing in intensity and number of needles as days go by. Massage may be tried.

In the *subacute phase*, after approximately 2 weeks, more active physiotherapy can be given. The physiotherapist performs a new examination concerning the range of movement and the muscular status. Mobilisation is instructed and performed with care, first free active movements and later turning, leaning and flexion movements against the resistance of the hand of the therapist. Bio-feedback training is helpful. This induces muscle strengthening enabling the patient to cease using the collar.

Now is also the time for treatment of other parts of the body. Thus the physician and the physiotherapist have to examine the range of movement in the cervical, thoracic and even the lumbar part of the spine, as thoracic as well as lumbar disturbances are common in traffic accidents together with neck lesions. Hypermobility and hypomobility are looked for. Asymmetries are noted.

Hypermobility is usually most common in the lumbar back, caused by the traffic trauma. Muscular stabilisation training is instructed and is usually the only treatment necessary.

Hypomobility is most common in the thoracic spine. The treatment is vertebral joint mobilisation.

In this stage it is of uttermost importance to induce leg muscle strength training, as for balance, walking, and returning to a normal life the use of the legs for appropriate stance and body support is mandatory. For the patients self-confidence one basic thing is the possibility to move around freely and be able with muscle power to counteract imbalances and not have to stop walking or training due to lack of leg muscle ability.

The sacroiliac joints are very important to examine after traffic accidents. The symptoms may be obscure and delayed in appearance. Sometimes symptoms and signs appear years after the trauma. The patient is examined standing up. Differences in height between the right and left iliac crests are looked for. The *Vorlauf* phenomenon, when one spina iliaca posterior is immobile when the patient bends forward, indicates immobility in one sacroiliac joint. The patient is treated according to the findings, with mobilisation of the immobile joint. This is performed with the patient in a lateral or prone position, the sacrum fixed and the iliac bone mobilised by the physiotherapist. Massage may help some patients considerably, but in others increase the pain.

In the *subchronic and chronic stage* more stabilisation training is performed, including neck movements with muscle strengthening. The training is performed, supervised and instructed by the physiotherapist and also with a written home training program. Video instructions are advisable. Both for neck training and general robustness of the whole body training in water is of benefit.

Most whiplash patients have balance problems caused by a brainstem disturbance or being of neck origin - cervical vertigo [3, 4]. Neck treatment may help, but often true balance training is needed: walking, turning, head and eye movements, standing on one leg, on a hubcap or on foam rubber [5, 6]. The automated training in the computerised forceplate, the Balance master, is of great help. The trauma may have caused benign positional paroxysmal vertigo, which craves a specific treatment [7].

The patient may be very tired and also have mental problems, with fatigue and depressive tendencies. Hence the psychological approach has to be considered by all members of the treating team, especially the physiotherapist who has a lot of contact with the patient, repeatedly and often in long sessions. The goal is to help the patient return to a normal family life and also to work.

Follow-Up

For the subsequent weeks, months, and even years it is of importance to have a well programmed follow-up of the whiplash patient. This should preferably be performed by the initial treatment team, who knows the patient and has participated in the assessment. The follow-up takes into consideration all angles of the problems, the neck, back, pelvis, and balance, as well as the psychological and practical problems. The treatment results are recorded by case history according to a questionnaire, and clinical investigation including balance testing. Stabilometry or, even better, dynamic posturography is performed for an objective assessment of the deficit and improvement in balancing ability.

The Whiplash Team

For handling patients with whiplash injuries a team of specialists is necessary. The members of different professions need special expertise concerning orthopedics, neurology, neck physiology and neuro-otology. The legal questions can best be answered by a physician in the whiplash team. The physiotherapist must have a profound knowledge of neck physiology and treatment, balance problems and vertigo. Education and information of physicians and physiotherapists are necessary to increase the awareness of the whiplash phenomenon, thereby preventing harmful delay in treatment and referral.

References

1. Mealy K, Brennan H, Fenelon GCC (1986) Early mobilisation of acute whiplash injuries. Br Med J 292:656-657
2. McKinney LA, Dornan JO, Ryan M (1989) The role of physiotherapy in the management of acute neck sprains following road-traffic accidents. Arch Emergency Med 6:27-33
3. Ålund M, Ledin T, Ödkvist LM, Larsson SE, Möller C (1993) Dynamic posturography among patients with common neck disorders. A study of 15 cases with suspected cervical vertigo. J Vestibular Res 3:383-389
4. Ålund M, Ledin T, Möller C, Odkvist LM, Larsson SE (1991) Dynamic posturography in cervical vertigo. Acta Otolaryngol, Stockh [Suppl 481]:601-602
5. Norré M, Beckers A (1988) Vestibular habituation training. Arch Otolaryngol Head Neck Surg 114:883-886
6. Ödkvist I, Ödkvist LM (1988) Physiotherapy in vertigo. Acta Otolaryngol, Stockh [Suppl 455]:74-76
7. Epley J (1992) The canalith reposition procedure: for treatment of benign paroxysmal vertigo. Otolaryngol Head Neck Surg 107:399-404

Neurorehabilitation of Ataxia

M. FORNI, E. ENOCK AND A. LINTURA

The meaning of ataxia is failure of coordination. Atactic patients are not able to define the width, velocity, and rhythms of muscle contractions, and cannot coordinate more muscle groups which are synchronously activated. The ataxia can be determined by: (1) injury of the proprioceptive afferences; (2) labyrinthic injury; (3) injury of cerebellum or its connections which are reciprocally connected to the cerebral cortex (neocerebellum), the spinal cord (paleocerebellum), and the vestibular system (archeocerebellum).

The walking ataxia - often generically considered as walking balance disease - can also be generated by an injury of the pyramidal paths causing an heavy recruitment deficit of the lower limb proximal areas.

We use the word "ataxia" with the meaning of coordination and motor control alteration due to the inability of the antagonistic muscle couples to synergistically operate. It can occur as postural instability of one or more body segments, or as dyssynergia when holding a posture during the execution of a complex motion [2, 6].

Ataxia can be often found in whiplash-type injuries and sometimes in the acute phase shows reversibility, probably because it is supported by a simple neuro-apraxia of the corresponding nervous paths.

In cases in which the ataxia is present with instability characteristics it is usually supported by injuries of the direct or indirect proprioceptive paths, or the cerebellospinal paths flowing to the cervical spinal cord.

From the functional point of view, ataxia can be defined as a specific difficulty in controlling the center of gravity of the whole body, or of single articulated segments. In fact, it magically disappears when the patient is immersed into water [3].

If considered on the plane of a system which can be influenced by therapeutic exercise, that is, on the interface between environment and spinal segmentary system (receptor level and muscle effector level), ataxia can be defined as the inability to couple suitably coactivation and reciprocal activation, the latter the pathologically prevalent characteristic.

From the spinal cord point of view, in fact, hypothonia could be consid-

Fondazione Don C. Gnocchi, Istituto di Marina di Massa (MS), Italy

ered as the cause of the ataxia. In fact, if we consider ataxia as increase of the stretching reflex threshold due to decreasing of the fusi basal discharge, we can formulate the hypothesis that the motion desynchronization is supported by a decreasing of the tonic "brake", due to perceptive distortions connected to the proprioceptor altered operation.

Further, we could consider ataxia as the extreme pole of a continuous path with variable prevalence grades between coactivation and reciprocal activation, in which the opposite is spasticity. In fact, correct motion requires a rigidity entity which is able to withstand stimuli, or a flexibility that is the ability to follow stimuli. Ataxia can be considered as an excessive flexibility. The posturogram of a normal person is known to often show variability in the centre of gravity displacement, which is the expression of physiologic flexibility. The motion pre-patterns, that is the anticipatory muscle activation of an intentional motion being carried out, are one of the physiological examples of the control of this CNS variability.

The therapeutic approach to ataxia cannot be separated from such considerations [4].

The most important problem in the spontaneous adaptation to the symptom in the atactic patient is normally that the spontaneous reaction increases the symptom.

The "body's intelligence" reacts against the instability by increasing the rigidity, that is the cocontraction, which is the real mechanism altered by the pathology. This condition activates the paradoxical happening so that the instability increases with the increasing of attempts aimed to limit it. Some preliminary therapeutical results can be obtained simply by disconnecting this vicious circle by means of relaxation techniques (which could be claimed as not suitable with regard to muscle tone assessment), also of the psychomotor type. Taking into consideration that often the whole spontaneous attempt of stopping the symptom accentuates it, the proposal of "balance exercises" for the atactic patient seems to be not justifiable. In fact, these exercises are based on quick changes of the centre of gravity, as imposed by the rehabilitator, and are also based on the idea that after some stress of this type an adaptation should occur. It is my opinion that this adaptation - based on the idea that the repetition is one of the mechanisms starting the process of learning - makes the ataxia problem not solvable from the rehabilitation point of view.

An exercise plan for the atactic patient should be based on a functional assessment, recognising the motion specific characteristics as well as the necessary changes needed to modify it. For example, we can examine whether the atactic motion is sensitive to inertial changes applied to the end of the considered segment (weights), or to intentional changes (automatic-voluntary dissociation), or even whether it uses any, and if so which, privileged afferent channels. Furthermore, the description of the altered motion should include the planes on which the alteration is mainly evident as well as the articular angles and motion velocity at which the motion is mainly compromised. Furthermore, we should examine whether the motion is dynamically or statically altered.

Clearly, the examiner's eye cannot record, not even summarily, the quantitative aspects. In many centres instrumental assessment involving dynamic (posturegraphy) and cinematic methods are being developed, as well as functional electromyography evaluations.

The traditional neurological vocabulary [7] does not offer the possibility to efficaciously describe the different clinic expressions of this disease, above all in terms of the therapy planning. The most interesting classification from the rehabilitation point of view is still P. Gasco's one [3], relevant to rehabilitation of motion in patients suffering from multiple sclerosis in its different expressions (Table 1).

Therefore we propose a descriptive assessment protocol to be associated, when possible, with instrumental evaluations [1, 5]:

1. Assessment of ataxia "migration" in different body areas, with reference to posture; in fact, often the oscillation of one segment is complementary to and compensates the adjacent segment oscillation and does not represent the injury site from the topological point of view. The patient is evaluated in different postures taking into consideration the syndrome's acuteness: for example, in the erect position (possibly also the monopodalic

Table 1. Correlations between lesions and symptoms

Lesion topography	Functions	Postural reactions	First order lesion associations	Second order lesion associations
Efferent motor paths	Pyramidal	Inhibited		
Posterior cord afferent paths	Kinesthesic and proprioceptive (deep sensory)	Uncompleted, delayed	With synergically reduced reactions	
Cerebro-cerebellar paths	Neo-cerebellar	Sequentially altered		With dissociated reactions
Spino-cerebellar paths	Paleo-cerebellar	Increased intensity		
Vestibulo-cerebellar paths	Archeo-cerebellar	Dynamically displaced with distal prevalence	With reactions uninhibited	
Vestibulo-spinal paths	Vestibular	Statically distorted with proximal prevalence	in direction and intensity	

position), both with extended and flexed knees, in a quadrupedic position, in crouched position, sitting down to exactly examine the planes at which the motion is more compromised, and the postural conditions in which the instability is evidenced in each body area. In the most difficult cases, the patient can also be evaluated in a supine position thanks to suitable supports able to allow the cingulum to move with one or more degrees of freedom.

2. Evaluation of synergies most stressed by the ataxia in the same body area [8]. Various modes of execution of the same action are evaluated (for example: reaching to a point in the space with one limb end or with the head, or tracking of a trajectory with one limb or the eyes, grasping of objects, reaching possible positions). In this phase, the performance success or the execution correctness is not evaluated, but the chosen "strategy", above all on the basis of the degrees of freedom or constraints imposed on the various segments implied or possible to be implied in the motion.

3. Evaluation of the maximal voluntary co-contraction effects on the symptoms [9]: the patient is asked to try to actively stop the tremor or the postural instability by stiffening as much as possible the involved segment and the adjacent segments. Under the same other conditions, we note cases in which this operation is successful and cases in which this operation causes instability or increasing incoordination.

4. Evaluation of differences in the symptoms with respect to the voluntariness or automatism of the motion; for example, in exercises with multiple conditions in which an upper limb is laid on a moving plane and executes automatic support functions, while the other limb executes an intentional job referred to a target imposed by the examiner; then the operation of the examined limbs is inverted. We note instability conditions which tend to occur more intentionally, than automatically, and vice versa (considering the required cautions due to the kinesiologic differences between the two tasks).

5. Evaluation of differences in the symptoms [10] subsequent to segmentary motions which are freely chosen by the patient, or segmentary motions imposed by the examiner, but without perceptive guide, or motions with perceptive guide, such as reaching a target or executing a trajectory following paths imposed by the examiner.

6. Evaluation of the effect of suppression, increase or distortion of one or more perceptive channels (acoustic, visual or proprioceptive) on the posture or motion.

The above six factors allow a functional assessment of the ataxia which is more suitable than the traditional one used to plan therapy. In this way, the therapeutic approach can be oriented to correction of the most specific aspects which determine the incoordination or balance deficiency.

204

Naturally, this approach should be widened and validated, if possible, with instrumental analysis able to control both the assessment correctness and the efficiency of the therapeutic approach.

To further this aim we are starting, together with the University of Pisa - Annexed Section of Neurorehabilitation - Prof. B. Rossi, an instrumental evaluation program supported by the ELITE system, which requires [11]:

1. Kinematic evaluations able to establish entity, velocity, acceleration of the angular displacements of different body segments as induced by the ataxia in different postures.
2. Dynamic (stabilometric) evaluations able to establish some characteristics of the body's or its segments' centre of gravity displacement in different postures.
3. Electromyographical evaluations which derive bioelectric activity contemporarily from four antagonist muscle couples of the lower limbs in an erect position and allow one to show, when present, the "cerebellar fall".

When it is not possible to adopt sophisticated instrumental evaluations, we think it is very useful to monitor the condition with videotapes, which can be associated with a functional assessment and allow one to have a relatively accurate idea about the efficiency of the treatment.

In the past, the rehabilitation treatment of ataxia has been applied through heavy and unuseful balance exercises, or through conditioning techniques whose technologic aspect has become more and more developed. For example, biofeedback is an instrument able to associate visual or acoustic stimuli to the patient's motion behaviour. These stimuli can increase the probability that under certain conditions a more suitable motion behaviour happens. The problem implied in the conditioning techniques is given by the short duration of the results and the performance dependence upon the associated stimulus.

An interesting perspective in ataxia therapy has been offered by the application of "perceptive conflict" exercises for treatment of feedback control deficiency. This approach, which can even use sophisticated methods such as virtual reality, is based on the importance given in the determination of ataxia to the perceptive aspect and to the possibility to restructure the balance system in the peripheral environment through induced perceptive alterations.

Another interesting attempt is the use of an EMG-acoustic device able to monitor muscular recruitment sequences in ballistic movements for treatment of pre-programming level. In addition, the technique known as kinematic muscle shortening with traction stress has also been successfully used. This method, based on quite new motor action organisation theories - the best known of which is A. Feldman's "equilibrium point" - is based on the possibility of recalling not present motion components, shortening a muscle when contemporarily a vibration is applied to the muscle itself (traction stress). In ataxia this exercise cannot be applied to all muscle groups; in fact, the associated hypotonia implies that the strengthening reaction is recalled at higher muscle lengths than the normal ones; sometime these lengths can exceed the articular limits of the considered segment. The muscles on which the exercise can be usually executed are short, generally phasic, muscle such as the posterior neck muscles, to which the head is suspended in the vertical posture. This exercise allowed us to obtain preliminary interesting results in head tremor control.

Other otoneurological techniques, almost of all which involve reflexo-logic imprinting, are exhaustively described in other reports.

In many serious cases it is possible to use technology to enable people with ataxia to perform intended tasks such as feeding themselves. There are three ways of reducing the effects of ataxia: (1) isolation from direct control; (2) modification of feedback; (3) mechanical loading for increasing inertia: by adding a spring with a definite stiffness, by adding mass, and by viscous damping.

Many damped orthoses have been created for many activities of daily living.

References

1. Andersen OT (1986) A system for quantitative assessment of dyscoordination and tremor. Acta Neurologica Scandinavica 73:291-294
2. Dietz HC et al (1992) The coordination of posture and voluntary movement in patients with cerebellar dysfunction. Movement Disorders 7(1):14-22
3. Gasco P (1994) La terapia riabilitativa dei pazienti con sclerosi multipla. In: Cazzullo et al (eds). Sclerosi Multipla. Masson, Milano
4. Grimaldi L et al (1986) Evocazione di componenti motorie assenti nelle lesioni del sistema nervoso centrale. II. Criteri di organizzazione degli atti motori. Giardini, Pisa
5. Hewer RL et al (1972) An investigation into the value of treating intention tremor by weighting the affected limb. Brain 95:579-590
6. Marsden CD (1975) The physiological basis of ataxia. Physiotherapy 61(11):326-328
7. Michaelis J (1993) Mechanical methods of controlling ataxia. In: Bailliere's (ed). Clinical Neurology. CD Ward
8. Morgan MH et al (1975) Intention tremor-a method of measurement. Journal of Neurology, Neurosurgery and Psychiatry 38:253-258
9. Sancesario G et al (1984) Fisiopatologia dei sintomi cerebellari. Riabilitazione e Apprendimento 4:59
10. Sanes JN et al (1988) Visual and mechanical control of postural and kinetic tremor in cerebellar system disorders. Journal of Neurology, Neurosurgery and Psychiatry 51:934-943
11. Tesio L et al (1992) Proposta di esercizio terapeutico per i disturbi motori nelle atassie. In: Atti del Corso di Aggiornamento "Le atassie ereditarie e le mioclono-epilessie", Courmayeur 1-4 aprile, 1992

Visual Feedback Center of Gravity Reeducation

D. Alpini, A. Cesarani[1] and M. De Bellis

Introduction

Maintaining postural stability is a complex process [10] involving the coordinated actions of biomechanical, sensory, motor, and central nervous system components. A relatively simple biomechanical definition for postural stability can be formulated in terms of the position of the body center of gravity relative to the base of support. The body movements used to maintain postural stability, however, are complex because of the number of joint systems and muscles involved. Sensing the position of the body relative to gravity and the base of support is also complex and involves combinations of visual, vestibular and somatosensory inputs [5, 6]. Central adaptive processes are required to modify the sensory and motor components so that stability can be maintained under a wide variety of task conditions.

The center of gravity (CoG) is the point at which the whole weight of a body may be considered to act. In humans who are standing quietly and vertically erect the CoG is located at the level of the hips and slightly forward of the ankle joints. CoG height is 0.5527 of total height. CoG and center of mass (CoM) are equivalent points in space when the gravitational field is uniform and gravity is the only force under consideration [7].

When the body moves about the ankles as a rigid mass (Fig. 1), vertically erect posture is observed when the CoG is directly over the center of feet support. In the AP direction, the center is halfway between the forward and backward boundaries of the support area. The body is vertically erect when the CoG is 14% of the foot length in front of the medial malleolus of the ankle joint. This alignment is equivalent to a baseline "forward lean" of the CoG of 2.3° with reference to an imaginary line passing through the ankle joints.

The Balance Master (Neurocom, Clackamas, OR, USA) is a piece of equip-

Ospedale Maggiore Policlinico, Istituto di Audiologia, Università degli Studi di Milano, Via Sforza 35, Milan, Italy
[1] ENT, Otoneurological Service Scientific Institute S. Maria N.te, F.ne don Gnocchi, Via Capecelatro 66, 20148 Milan, Italy

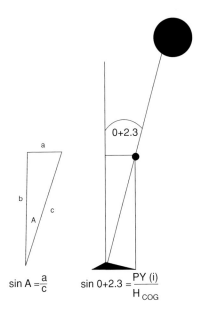

$$\sin A = \frac{a}{c} \qquad \sin 0+2.3 = \frac{PY\ (i)}{H_{COG}}$$

Fig. 1. Geometric relationship between θ *(i)* and PY *(i)*

ment that allows, by means of a dual footplate, a visual feedback of CoG position, projected on a computer screen facing the patient standing on the platform. It allows either diagnostic posturographic assessments or equilibrium training based on visual feedback. The static diagnostic tasks involve minimization of standing postural sway under three conditions: eyes open, eyes closed, eyes open with visual feedback.

The Balance Master presents the therapist and the patient with a comprehensive program of balance rehabilitation [3, 4, 9]. It has the capability for both quantitative assessment and training.

Balance Master Principles of Operation

The Balance master footplate consists of two 9-inch footplates [11]. There is a pin joint between the two plates, 9 inches from the rear border of the plates. The axis along the pin joint constitutes the X (lateral) axis. The pin joint also intersects the Y (anteroposterior axis).

Each footplate rests on two force transducers with the sensitive axes oriented vertically. The transducers are mounted along the front-to-back center line of each plate (one 8.25 inches behind and the other 8.125 inches in front of the pin joint). The lateral distance between left and right plate transducers and center is 5.00 inches (Fig. 2).

The sum of the vertical forces exerted on the left footplate transducers is equal to the sum of forces on the right footplate transducers when the vertical force center is located at any point along the boundary between the two plates. This places the X axis zero position at the Y axis.

For each footplate, the vertical forces exerted on the front and the back transducers are equal when the vertical forces exerted on the plate are centered between the front and back transducers (i.e. at the pin joint). This places the Y axis zero position at the pin joint.

The total vertical force exerted on the two foot plates is calculated by summing the four vertical force signals. Antero-posterior CoG sway angle is the angle between a vertical line projecting upward from the center of the area of feet support and a second line projecting from the same point to the subject's CoG. When normal subjects maintain a vertically erect position, the CoG is located directly over the area of the feet support, slightly forward of the ankle joints. This position can be maintained without stepping or reaching for support if sway does not exceed the subject's limits of stability (Fig. 3).

In theory, the forward limit of stability places the CoG over the front boundary of the support area; the backward stability limit places the CoG over the back boundary of the support area. In practice, the effective limits of stability are somewhat smaller than would be predicted by foot length, since in most individuals the strength of the intrinsic foot muscles prevents the bearing of the full body weight by the toes or the extreme back of the heel.

Functional stability limits have been calculated [10] to be 6.25° anteriorly and 4.45° posteriorly for the average adult subject. The angular limits of stability are very nearly the same for all adults regardless of height.

When a subject is standing quietly on the Balance Master forceplate with ankles placed symmetrically over the electrical center of the forceplate, the vertical projection of CoG is assumed to intersect the forceplate at the center of the vertical force position. As the body moves more rapidly, the vertical projection of the CoG lags increasingly behind the center of vertical force.

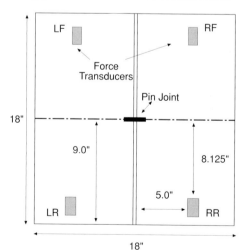

Fig. 2. Forceplate configuration

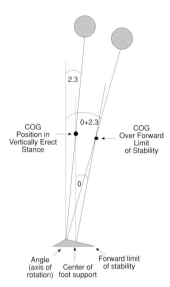

Fig. 3. Center of gravity sway angle and stability limits

When CoG sway is a reflection of the body rotating as a rigid mass about the ankle joints, there are no horizontal components of force exerted against the support surface. In contrast, hip movement generates horizontal forces against the support surface that are proportional to the acceleration of the hip joint angle. Changes in vertical force position during hip movement only occur when hip movement also causes changes in the CoG sway angle.

Planning the Treatment: The Limits of Stability Test

To maintain stability with the feet in place, the body's CoG must be positioned vertically over the base of support. When this condition is met, a person can both resist the destabilizing influence of gravity and actively move the CoG. If the CoG is positioned outside the perimeter of the base of support, the person has exceeded the in-place limits of stability. At this point, to prevent a fall, a rapid step or stumble to reestablish the base of support beneath the CoG or additional external support is required.

The base of support for standing on a flat, firm surface is defined as the area contained within the perimeter of contact between the surface and the two feet. The base of support area is nearly square when the feet are placed comfortably apart during quiet standing.

The limits of stability (LoS) measure is a two-dimensional quantity defining the largest possible CoG sway angle as a function of sway direction from the center position. The LoS depends on the placement of the feet and the base of support. In normal adults standing on a flat, firm surface with feet comfortably apart, the LoS perimeter can best be described as an ellipse. The AP dimension of this ellipse is approximately $12.5°$ from the most backward point to the most forward point on the perimeter. Although height of the CoG above the surface and the foot length affect the AP limits of stability, these two features covary, resulting in approximately the same AP limits for persons of various heights. The lateral LoS depends on the person's height relative to the spacing between the feet. When the feet of a person 180 cm tall are placed 10 cm apart, for example, the lateral dimension of the LoS ellipse is approximately $16°$ from the farthest point on the left to the farthest point on the right of the perimeter.

The biomechanical properties that determine the LoS are similar for standing in place, walking, and sitting without trunk support. During in-place standing the CoG moves randomly within an LoS perimeter determined by the base of support and the placement of the feet. During walking the CoG progresses forward through the LoS in a smooth rythmic movement. At heel strike an LoS is established with the CoG positioned at the posterior perimeter. As the step progresses, the CoG moves forward within the LoS. As the CoG approaches the anterior perimeter of the LoS, the next step establishes a new LoS and the rhythmic process is repeated. When a person is sitting without trunk support the height of the CoG above the support surface is lower and the base area is larger. Therefore the LoS perimeter is larger when a person is seated than during quiet standing.

For these reasons re-education of the limits of stability in standing in place can be used to rehabilitate the patient to regain normal LoS during walking, too.

When a person's postural stability is disrupted by an external perturbation (in whiplash patients it can be even the gravity force), one or a combination of three different strategies is typically used to coordinate movement of the CoG back to a balanced position. When body displacement is beyond the LoS perimeter, a step or stumbling reaction is the only movement strategy effective in preventing fall. When the CoG remains within the LoS, two different strategies or combination thereof can be used to move the CoG while maintaining the initial placement of the feet on the support surface: the ankle strategy and the hip strategy. The correct execution of the LoS test requires normal combined and integrated ankle-hip strategies. The relative effectiveness of these two kind of postural strategies in positioning and maintaining the CoG in the desired position (Fig. 5) depends on the configuration of the base of support, the CoG alignment in relation to the LoS, and the speed of the postural movement [8, 12, 15].

A normal individual moves primarily about the ankles when sway amplitudes are well within the LoS and increases the use of hip movement when sway approaches the LoS. Postural movements are ineffective in the patient who uses ankle strategy movements to control sway displacements of large amplitude. The patient who depends on ankle movements falls prematurely when sway amplitudes are large. The patient using hip movements to control sway of small amplitude is inefficient and expends a needlessly high level of energy to maintain a centered CoG position. Ineffective use of movements strategies may be caused by abnormal adaptation or by an inability to produce one of the two movement patterns; for example, inappropriate use of the hip movements during sway of small amplitude caused by anxiety or by misperception of the LoS. Anxiety and LoS misperception are common findings in whiplash patients. In these cases training aimed at teaching the appropriate conditions for using ankle movements can have a positive impact. In contrast, weakness of ankle joint muscles, loss of ankle sensation, reduced mobility about the ankles, or combinations of these factors prevent the patient from generating effective ankle movements and might be an abnormal adaptation used by a dizzy patient to minimize head movements and associated stimulation of the neck and vestibular system. Di Fabio and Andersen [2] showed, in fact, that a distortion of the somatosensory inputs from the ankles altered the displacement of the head whether the eyes were open or closed, and visual information is necessary to coordinate specific postural patterns utilizing horizontal shear forces to maintain stance on a mechanically compliant surface. The control of the head position during balance is also dependent on somatosensory inputs from the feet or lower limbs which are generated by foot contact with the supporting surface.

Shumway-Cook et al. [14] conducted the first study that used objective visual feedback, based on symmetry of postural sway (movement of the CoG), for training purposes. This study compared the effectiveness of visual feedback to more conventional physical therapy techniques for reestablishing symmetry of standing in hemiparetic patients. During sessions, the therapist also gave tactile and verbal cues to assist patients in maintaining good postural alignment [13];

The LoS test is a dynamic task that requires voluntary sway, as accurately as possible, toward eight visual targets sequentially lighted up on a computer screen. Feedback indicating the location of the subject's own CoG is visible on the screen during all the tests and during the further training [1].

The LoS test is a "two tailed test", in which the best performance is in the middle of the scale, and the "worst" performances are at the top and the bottom of the scale. In this test the goal is to put the cursor in the center of the target. Staying at the target is good; undershooting the target is bad and overshooting the target is bad, too. The bell curve for this type of test, referred to a normative population, will have two tails. A rank of 2.5% or lower is abnormal. A rank of 97.5% or higher is abnormal. Ranks between 2.5% and 97.5% are normal. So a patient with a rank in the 4th percentile (4%) on a two-tailed test is considered normal for that test (Fig. 4).

212

Balance Master diagnostic values are expressed referring patient perform-ance to normative data (according to age and height). Normative data are graphically reported according to a percentile scale that is not linear. It is instead logarithmic so that the abnormal range is magnified in order to better distinguish slightly abnormal from very abnormal (Fig. 5).

The data is analyzed only for movement away from the center. After the cue moves to the highlighted target, the patient will be measured for 8 s. The subject must reach the target within 4 s to get a set of scores that can all be compared to normative data.

The LoS test informs regarding the ability to move to different points in space and remain stable there, critical for normal motor function. High tar-get sway scores indicate instability at those points in space.

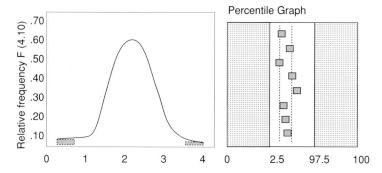

Fig. 4. Double-tail graph: *darkened areas* indicate the outside 5%, 2.5% on each side

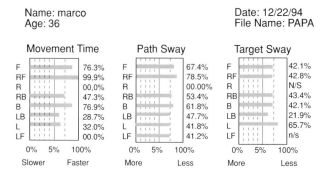

Fig. 5. Example of normative percentile representation of LoS test

Treatment

The LoS test records for 8 s, 4 of which are given for transit time. The last 4 s are used to collect target sway data.

On the LoS test the "movement time" score tells (Fig. 6) how many seconds it took to reach the desired target. It does not tell about reaction time so that it cannot be determined whether a high score reflects a delay in response time followed by slow movements or a combination of slow reaction time and slow movement.

The "path sway" refers percentage of path length.

The "target sway" is expressed as percentage of maximum CoG area maintained on the target.

The "patient position" value is given in polar coordinates and represents the average position of the CoG during the period of target sway assessment. If the target was not reached, the patient position score reflects the point of closest approach to the target.

PATIENT INFORMATION AND TEST SETTINGS

Patient Name:	Age: 30	Test Date. 02/16/95
Data file	Ht.: 172 cm	Order #:6
Target/prot. Type: SP06	LOS: 75%	Pacing Speed: 10 sec.
Therapy Mode: Beep, Feedback		
Post-Test Comment:		

Limits of stability

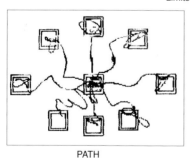
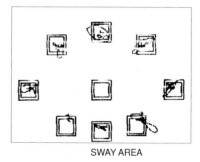

PATH   SWAY AREA

Numeric Summary

Transition		Mvt Time (sec)	Path Sway (% Path Len)	Target Sway (% Max Area)	Patient Position (% LOS)	(deg)	Distance Error (% LOS)	Direction Error (deg)
1	(F)	4.28	127.68	N/S	<72.1>	<359.2>	<-2.9>	<-0.8>
2	(RF)	4.00	172.16	0.41	70.8	42.7	-4.2	-2.3
3	(R)	4.04	157.96	N/S	<71.8>	<87.8>	<-3.2>	<-2.2>
4	(RB)	2.94	169.83	0.58	68.6	124.8	-6.4	-10.2
5	(B)	3.74	237.19	0.13	66.8	176.6	-8.2	-3.4
6	(LB)	6.72	347.19	N/S	<60.6>	<230.8>	<-14.4>	<-5.8>
7	(L)	4.50	188.06	N/S	<73.4>	<271.9>	<-1.6>	<1.9>
8	(LF)	3.70	158.90	0.20	70.1	314.2	-4.9	-0.8

Fig. 6. Example of LoS, a not completely statistical representation

The "distance error" is given as percent LoS and it is the difference between the patient's average position and the center of target. This parameter allows one to see how far away from the center the patient is willing and able to move in a given direction. A negative sign in front of the distance error number means the target was undershot; a positive number means a target was overshot.

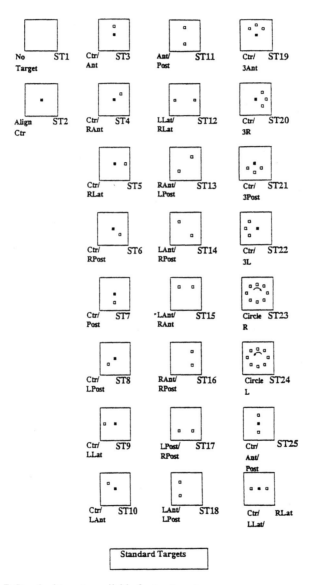

Fig. 7. Standard targets available for treatment

Even if the patient cannot reach the targets at the set LoS, the patient position (point of closest approach) can be used as a baseline to set target distance in exercise or training.

The direction error is given in degrees and it is the difference between the patient's average position and the center of the target. It allows one to see how far clockwise or counter-clockwise from the center of the target the patient held themselves. A negative sign in front of the direction error means the error was in a counter-clockwise direction; a positive number means the error was in a clockwise direction.

Distance error and direction error reflect the accuracy with which the target was achieved. Small error numbers mean greater accuracy.

By means of the Balance Master it is possible to treat patients ranging from 76 to 203 cm in height and from 18 to 138 kg in weight.

On the basis of the LoS test results one or more training programs is chosen out of the 26 standard targets (Fig. 7). Each treatment session can be performed according to the LoS, ranging from 25% to 100% of the predictable LoS, in 5% increments. The target pacing is 1, 3, 5, 7, 10, 15, 20 s. If trying to promote faster movement, then low pacing settings (1, 2, 5 s) are appropriate, such as in the case shown in Fig. 8. If stability at points in space is desired, then higher pacing settings (10 s or higher) are appropriate so that the patient must "hold" a position.

Figures 9-11 refer to a 30 year old patient suffering from dizziness 3 months after a whiplash injury. In Fig. 9 the pathological values are indicated in brackets, while in Fig. 10 the same pathological values are indicated by a dark column and referred to in percentiles. In this patient the LoS test shows that there are problems in maintaining correct equilibrium forward strategies, regarding time and path sway, right forward regarding movement time and target sway, and left forward regarding movement time and target sway. Figure 11 shows that there is not significant dysmetria (only a slight tendency to overshoot) and that endpoint direction error is not constantly clockwise or counter-clockwise.

In Fig. 12 the planned training program is shown. Because other tests indicate a right vestibulo-spinal deficit we prefered to train the patient only with right targets, with a medium pacing (10 s) to allow precise movements and well maintained positions. An acoustic (beep) feedback was introduced in order to improve reactions and movement times.

Figures 13 and 14 refer to a 50 year old patient suffering from instability and transient positional and positioning vertigo 8 months after the whiplash. Figure 13 shows difficulties in forward and right back movement times, right back and left path sway, forward and right back target sway. Figure 14 shows no preference in clockwise or counter-clockwise endpoint direction errors and no dysmetrias.

Figure 15 shows the chosen training program. In the first session of treat-

Balance Master: Analysis of Results
Comparision to Clinically Normal Scores

Dynamic Balance at 75% Limits of Stability
In 8 Movements Directions
F = Front B = Back L = Left R = Right

Name: Date: 02/16/95
Age: 30   File Name:

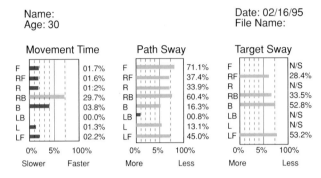

Movement Time		Path Sway		Target Sway	
F	01.7%	F	71.1%	F	N/S
RF	01.6%	RF	37.4%	RF	28.4%
R	01:2%	R	33.9%	R	N/S
RB	29.7%	RB	60.4%	RB	33.5%
B	03.8%	B	16.3%	B	52.8%
LB	00.0%	LB	00.8%	LB	N/S
L	01.3%	L	13.1%	L	N/S
LF	02.2%	LF	45.0%	LF	53.2%

0% 5% 100%   0% 5% 100%   0% 5% 100%
Slower   Faster   More   Less   More   Less

Fig. 8. Example of pathological LoS test at low pacing

9   PATIENT INFORMATION AND TEST SETTINGS

Patient Name: nicoletta   Age: 30   Test Date. 02/16/95
Data file   Ht.:   Order #:6
Target/prot. Type: SP06   LOS: 75%   Pacing Speed: 10 sec.
Therapy Mode: Beep, Feedback
Post-Test Comment:

Limits of stability

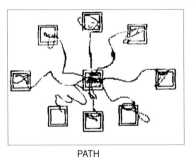 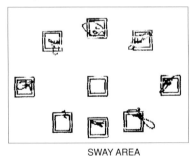

PATH   SWAY AREA

Numeric Summary

Transition		Mvt Time (sec)	Path Sway (% Path Len)	Target Sway (% Max Area)	Patient Position (% LOS)	(deg)	Distance Error (% LOS)	Direction Error (deg)
1	(F)	3.68	207.81	0.05	71.9	358.7	-3.1	-1.3
2	(RF)	4.42	158.83	N/S	<77.6>	<42.8>	<2.6>	<2.2>
3	(R)	3.74	159.71	0.08	73.0	88.0	-2.0	-2.0
4	(RB)	2.14	222.60	0.04	72.7	135.5	-2.3	0.5
5	(B)	2.52	240.30	0.23	70.1	175.5	-4.9	-4.5
6	(LB)	2.28	162.61	0.17	69.7	226.8	-5.3	1.8
7	(L)	3.62	183.18	0.09	68.3	272.8	-6.7	2.8
8	(LF)	4.02	169.01	N/S	<74.2>	<315.6>	<-0.8>	<0.6>

Balance Master: Analysis of Results
Comparision to Clinically Normal Scores

10

Dynamic Balance at 75% Limits of Stability
In 8 Movements Directions
F = Front B = Back L = Left R = Right

Name:
Age: 30

Date: 02/16/95
File Name:

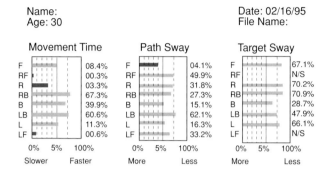

Balance Master: Analysis of Results
Comparision to Clinically Normal Scores

11

Dynamic Balance at 75% Limits of Stability
In 8 Movements Directions
F = Front B = Back L = Left R = Right

Name:
Age: 30

Date: 02/16/95
File Name:

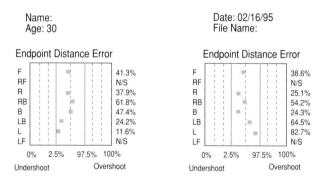

Figs. 9-11. Representation of LoS test in a 30 year old patient suffering from dizziness 3 months after a whiplash injury. **Fig. 9.** The pathological values are indicated in *brackets*. **Fig. 10.** The same pathological values are indicated by the *dark column* and refer to percentiles such as shown in Fig. 5

ment the movement time and path sway are correct (the time pacing is 5 s) while all the data referring to target sway are incorrect. Figure 16 shows the modified training program. The targets are the same as in the previous figure but the time pacing is 15 s in order to allow the patient to reach and maintain the correct target position. No acoustic feedback was provided.

Regarding Balance Master training, the duration of each session treatment is 20 min. The frequence generally varies from twice a week to every

PATIENT INFORMATION AND TEST SETTINGS

Patient Name: Age: 30   Test Date. 02/16/95
Data file   Ht.: 160 cm   Order #:4
Target/prot. Type: ST20   LOS: 75%   Pacing Speed: 10 sec.
Therapy Mode: Feedback
Post-Test Comment:

20 Ctr/3R

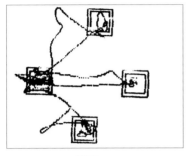
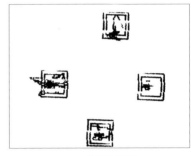

PATH   SWAY AREA

Numeric Summary

Transition	Mvt Time (sec)	Path Sway (% Path Len)	Target Sway (% Max Area)	Patient Position (% LOS)	Patient Position (deg)	Distance Error (% LOS)	Direction Error (deg)
1	4.98	182.15	0.27	70.4	47.4	-4.6	2.4
2	2.74	116.52	0.26	1.4	347.3	1.4	-12.7
3	3.88	121.11	0.04	72.4	89.2	-2.6	-0.8
4	2.70	106.98	0.28	2.6	316.0	2.6	-44.0
5	3.68	214.54	0.18	76.0	135.9	1.1	0.9
6	2.22	122.02	0.25	3.2	272.8	3.2	-87.2

Fig. 12. The numeric values of the proposed exercise

day treatment. The frequence of training sessions is dependent on a combination of other rehabilitative treatments such as physical therapy and vestibular electrical stimulation.

Conclusions

Visual feedback provides a ready source of information about postural instability for both the patient and the therapist. The purpose of Balance Master is to detect and make available to the patient objective information about physiological function or movement that is not ordinarily perceived by the patient. In the case of postural instability caused by whiplash injuries, visual, and auditory (beep), signals have been used to give the patient information about head and trunk orientation and about symmetry of weight bearing through the lower extremities. The assumption is that the patient can use visual or auditory cues better than he or she could use somatosensory or vestibular inputs.

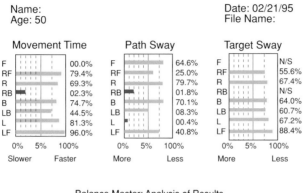

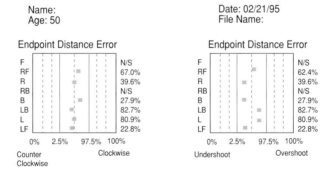

Figs. 13, 14. Representation of LoS test in a 50 year old patient suffering from instability and transient postonal and positioning vertigo 8 months after the whiplash

For the therapist the Balance Master establishes a baseline of patient function, facilitates the design of custom treatments, and evaluates the effectiveness of the therapeutic program.

For the patient it enhances motivation through real-time visual feedback, links perception to movement, internalizes the appropriate alignment or movement pattern, improves volitional control, and builds confidence to perform activities of daily living.

220

Patient Name: maria rosa   Age: 50   Test Date. 02/21/95
Data file   Ht.: 149 cm   Order #:5
Target/prot. Type: ST21   LOS: 75%   Pacing Speed: 5 sec.
Therapy Mode: Feedback
Post-Test Comment: 5 secondi

21: Cir/3Po

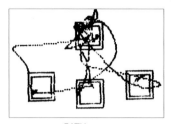 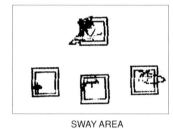

PATH   SWAY AREA

Numeric Summary

Transition	Mvt Time (sec)	Path Sway (% Path Len)	Target Sway (% Max Area)	Patient Position (% LOS)	Patient Position (deg)	Distance Error (% LOS)	Direction Error (deg)
1	1.44	124.22	N/S	<71.5>	<130.8>	<-3.3>	<-4.2>
2	1.70	111.02	N/S	<6.7>	<299.6>	<6.7>	<-60.4>
3	1.28	120.97	N/S	<66.5>	<183.3>	<-8.4>	<3.3>
4	1.88	122.30	N/S	<8.5>	<319.6>	<8.5>	<-40.4>
5	2.66	226.74	N/S	<83.0>	<226.4>	<8.2>	<1.4>
6	3.40	210.19	N/S	<13.6>	<241.8>	<13.6>	<-118.2>

Fig. 15. The numeric values of the proposed exercise

BALANCE MASTER

training

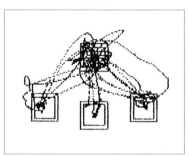

PATH

Fig. 16. The same exercise as in Fig. 15
performed at 15 s pace timing

References

1. Daleiden S (1990) Weight shifting as a treatment for balance deficits. A literature review. Physiother Can 48:81-87
2. Di Fabio RP, Andersen JH (1993) Effect of sway-referenced visual and somatosensory inputs on human head movement and postural patterns during stance. J Vest Res 3:409-417
3. Hamann KF, Krausen C (1990) Clinical application of posturography. Body tracking and biofeedback training. In: Brandt T, Paulus W, Bles W (eds). Disorders of Posture and Gait. Thieme, Stuttgart, 295-298
4. Hamann R, Panzer V, Mekjavic I (1992) A comparison of postural therapeutic regimens using visual feedback of the center of gravity. In: Wollacott M, Horak F (eds). Posture and gait. Control mechanisms, vol II, Eugene, University of Oregon, Books, 376-379
5. Hinoki M, Hine S, Okada S, Ishida Y, Koike S, Shizuku S (1975) Optic organ and cervical prorpioceptors in maintenance of body equilibrium. Acta Otolaryngol [Suppl 330]:169-184
6. Hinoki M, Ushio N (1975) Lumbomuscular proprioceptive reflexes in body equilibrium. Acta Otolaryngol [Suppl 330]:197-210
7. Horstmann GA, Dietz V (1990) A basic control mechanism: the stabilization of the center of gravity. Electroenceph Clin Neurophysiol 76:165-176
8. Lee DN, Lishman JR (1975) Visual proprioceptive control of stance. J Hum Mov Stud 1:87
9. Moore S, Wollacott MH (1993) The use of Biofeedback devices to improve postural stability. Phys Ther Pract 2(2):1-19
10. Nashner L (1994) Evaluation of postural stability, movement, and control. In: Hasson SM (ed). Clinical exercise physiology. Mosby, St Louis, p 57
11. Neurocom International Inc. Balance Master Operator's Manual. Portland Or, Neurocom, 1989
12. Previc FH (1992) The effects of dynamic visual stimulation on perception and motor control. J Vest Res 2:285-295
13. Paulus WM, Straube A, Brandt Th (1984) Visual stabilization of posture: physiological stimulus characteristics and clinical aspects. Brain 107:1143
14. Shumway-Cook A, McCollum G (1991) Assessment and treatment of balance deficits in the neurologic patients. In: Montgomery P, Connelly B (eds). Motor Control. Theoretical framework and parctical application to physical therapy. Chattanooga, Tn, Chattanooga Corp, 123-138
15. Ushio N, Hinoki M, Nakanishi K, Baron JB (1680) Role des propriocepteurs des muscles oculaires dans le maintain de l'équilibre du corps avec reference notamment au reflee cervical. Aggressologie 21:143-152

Ski Trainer Oscillating Platform: Proprioceptive Reeducation

M. Savini, D. Alpini and A. Cesarani [1]

Reeducation of the proprioceptive reflexes is especially indicated in post-traumatic disequilibrium. This method uses the theoretical premises of the method known as "proprioceptive neuromuscular facilitation" by: (1) the use of nervous information of surface origin (tactile data); (2) coordination of the information of deep origin (joint place, stretching of tendons and capsuloligamentous complexes.

This peripheral information stimulates the nervous system, which triggers the muscle. In this way the patient may relearn to balance on his foot or knee via recoordination of the reflexes in unstable positions. He thus learns progressively to admit and understand the unstableness after an accident and is guided to fight against this residual unstableness through a improved muscular interplay.

Skitter is a ski trainer platform comprised of an oscillating plate on which two foot pads are placed. Each foot pad is able to move antero-posteriorly (toes up and toes down) and lateral senses also allow torsional movement of each foot. The plate on which the two foot pads are placed is able to surf on an oscillating small table (Fig. 1). The oscillations of the table are slowed by elastic cords that regulate the resistence with which the device opposes the patient's movements. These movements of the feet and especially, surfing and oscillating of the body simulate the movements performed during skiing (Fig. 2).

Some exercises on Skitter were proposed either for sport training or for fitness. We usually employed Skitter for proprioceptive reeducation of post-traumatic unsteadiness and dizziness because it allows the use of cognitively involved exercises and improvement of sensorial coordination when visual feed-back is associated.

To successfully reeducate reflexes by this method, active cooperation of the subject is needed. The careful activity of a re-educator or of a physiotherapist offers better chances of success.

In whiplash patients we standardized a protocol that has been used in

Center for Vertigo Treatment, Hospital S. Rita, Via Catalani 20, Milan
[1] Institute of Audiology, University of Milan, Via F. Sforza 35, Milan

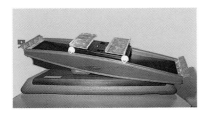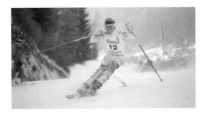

Figs. 1, 2. Skitter and skier

patients ranging from 18 to 45 years of age. According to the obvious limits of age, Skitter can be employed (with the constant help of the reeducator) also in older subjects, but usually it is not possible to perform the entire protocol. To achieve a good result, it is crucial that the articulations of ankle, knee and hip are complete and that the muscular tone, especially of the thigh, is good. Sometimes previous tonification of the muscles is in fact necessary before starting reeducation of the proprioceptive reflexes.

Forward leg extensions (Fig. 3):
1. With one foot on the end cap and the other across the foot pad, the patient keeps his weight forward and extends the front leg in a controlled manner, then he returns slowly and repeats. It improves quads and trunk muscles and stabilizes ankles and knees.
2. The patient maintains the leg extension position and the therapist destabilizes him by moving the platform during visual fixation of a point.
3. The patient performs a leg extension with closed eyes to improve self-perception of muscle tone.

Backward leg extensions (Fig. 4):
This is similar to forward leg extensions except the focus is on the rear leg. With a stable, controlled movement, the patient extends the leg back to the end and repeats on both legs. It improves gluts and quads, hamstrings and trunk muscles and stabilizes ankles and knees.

According to the neuro-otologic and equilibriometric characteristics of the patient, leg extensions should be performed for both legs or only for one leg.

Ankle-hip strategies (Fig. 5):
The patient steps on the foot pads with feet centrally positioned. Then he concentrates on proper posture using a mirror to see his reflection and transfers his weight from one foot to the other with a smooth flowing motion. During this smooth and rythmic weight transfer the therapist induces body movements according to ankle or hip strategies.

224

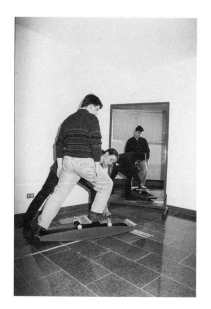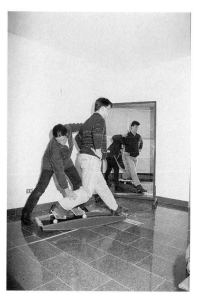

Fig. 3, 4. Forward (3) and backward (4) leg extensions

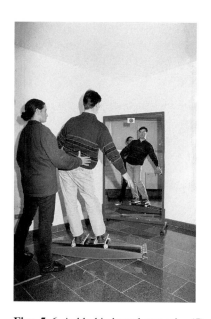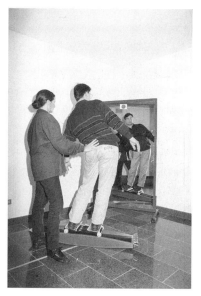

Figs. 5, 6. Ankle-hip lateral strategies (5) and with oscillations (6)

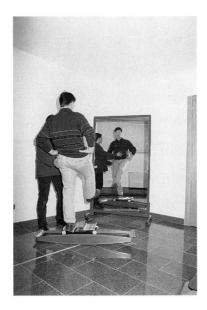 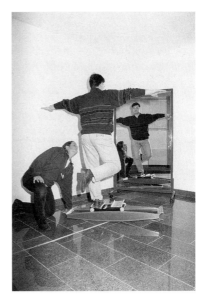

Figs. 7, 8. Extended **(7)** or flexed **(8)** exercises with one leg

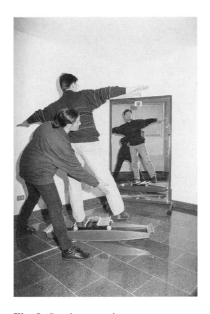 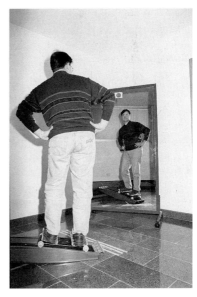

Fig. 9. One leg exercise   **Fig. 10.** Slalom exercise

Visual Feedback:
The patient is comfortably stable on the foot pads. With his thumbs and extended limbs he tries to touch some visual targets placed in different positions on a mirror in front of him.

Oscillations (Fig. 6):
The patient steps on foot pads with feet centrally positioned. Then he concentrates on proper posture using a mirror to see his reflection. With eyes closed he transfers his weight from one foot to the other with a smooth flowing motion. During this smooth and rythmic weight transfer the therapist pushes the bumpers at one end of the Skitter inducing a sudden and unpredictable inclination of the device.

One leg:
The patient maintains equilibrium on one leg with the other extended (Fig. 7) or flexed (Fig. 8) or with one leg lateral (Fig. 9). The therapist helps the patient either to maintain equilibrium or to correct his posture. A mirror facilitates postural equilibrium strategies correction.

Slalom (Fig. 10):
The patient steps on the foot pads with feet centrally positioned. Then he concentrates on proper posture using a mirror to see his reflection and begins to transfer his weight from one foot to the other with a smooth flowing motion. As his rythms increase he will get closer to the bumpers at each end, always maintaining good upright posture with eyes focused in the mirror and paying attention to his balance. If the exercise is performed with limited upper body movement (such as in slalom) it improves hip rotators, quads and calves, while it stimulates abdominal stabilizers and gluts when the patient includes upper body motion (such as in giant slalom). Exercises have to be performed concentrating on proper edge setting techniques.

Ankles stability:
The patient keeps his knees straight pushing the skate forward with his toes and pulling back with his heels. He has to concentrate on using only the ankles and calves, while all the other muscles are relaxed. It improves calves and ankle stability and balance proprioception.

Vestibular Electrical Stimulation

A. Cesarani and D. Alpini[1]

Proprioceptive Projections from the Neck to the Vestibular Nuclei

Peripheral proprioceptors of the muscles and the joints have a feedback control on the vestibular nuclei through spino-vestibular pathways. Neuromuscular spindles and Golgi receptors are dynamometers and they are particularly sensitive to variations in muscle length and tension. Joint receptors, Ruffini and Golgi bodies give information regarding the position of a joint and its movement. The portion of the neck including the first three vertebrae is particularly involved during the major part of everyday head movements. The paravertebral muscles of this region are very rich in proprioceptors. They are especially concentrated in the splenius capitis, the rectus capitis major, the longissimus capitis and the semispinalis capitis. These muscles comprise the deep plane of the nuchal muscles. The splenius is more superficial. The muscles act in the extension of homolateral bending and rotation of the head. During head movements they discharge to the vestibular nuclei [16, 17, 33].

Corbin and Hinsey [14] described direct projection from the first three cervical roots to the inferior vestibular nucleus. Fredrikson [15] showed the convergence of cervical and labyrinthine inputs on vestibular nuclei.

Hikosaka and Maeda [19] pointed out that the convergence especially involved inputs from the horizontal semicircular canal: the electrical stimulation of the vestibular nerve induces action potentials in the controlateral abducens nerve. This response is increased when also neck roots are contemporarily stimulated. The authors stated that there is facilitatory convergence of proprioceptive inputs from C2-C3 receptors on the medial vestibular nucleus of the opposite side and an inhibition on the ipsilateral muscles. The latency between electrical stimulation of the dorsal cervical roots and vestibular nucleus response is only 2 ms. The authors thus hypothesized direct projections from neck to vestibular nuclei.

Ospedale Maggiore Policlinico, Istituto di Audiologia, Università degli Studi di Milano, Via Sforza 35, Milan, Italy
[1] ENT, Otoneurological Service Scientific Institute S. Maria N.te, F.ne don Gnocchi, Via Capecelatro 66, 20148 Milan, Italy

228

Maeda [28] described proprioceptive nuchal afferences on the Schwalbe nucleus.

Boyle and Pompeiano [5] showed that neurons in the dorso-caudal portion of the Deiter's nucleus receive tonic cervical inputs while the neurons in the rostro-ventralis portion receive especially otolithic inputs.

Raymond and Sans [31] demonstrated that Roller's nucleus and the accessory group Y receive ipsilateral projections from the cervical mucles.

Wilson [34] described cerebellar projections on the nodulus and the flocculus, while Berthoz and Llinas [2] described projections on the cerebellar anterior lobus.

Mergner at al. [29] demonstrated proprioceptive convergences in 80% of the neurons in the suprasilvian parietal cortical vestibular area. Sensitive inputs run through IA and IIA fibers that run along spinal cord and through the spino-reticular and spino-cerebellar fasciculus that seem to send direct projections to the vestibular nuclei.

Vibration of the Neck

The vibration of muscles or muscle tendons alters proprioceptive input and produces kinesthetic illusions in human subjects.

A lot of clinical and experimental evidence exists regarding the effects of vibration of the paravertebral muscles on posture control and head-trunk coordination. Generally the effects are based on the activation of the cervico-spinal reflexes (CSRs): bending the neck and turning the head relative to the body evokes reflexes in the limb muscles either in decerebrate cats [2, 4, 25] or in human beings [18, 20, 22, 27].

These reflexes interact with vestibulo-spinal reflexes (VSRs) controlling extensory muscle tone. Vestibular and proprioceptive inputs are integrated either in Deiter's vestibular nucleus or in the nucleo-reticular formation. Proprioceptive inputs are generated in muscle spindles of the neck muscles and are partially responsible for the elicitation of CSRs.

It is known [21, 23] that it is possible, in the absence of any actual movement, to induce kinesthetic illusions and associated motor responses in humans when mechanical vibrations are applied either to the distal tendon of a limb muscle or to the neck [24, 26, 32]. Illusory movements and/or motor responses can be extended the the whole body when vibrations are applied to muscles involved in postural stance, such as neck muscles.

Vibration therefore constitutes an efficient means of obtaining true copies of actual sensory messages and thus of eliciting "at will" illusory movements the direction, speed and duration of which can be preselected.

Vibration of the posterior muscles of the neck has been shown to induce illusions of changed position and of motion of a visual target when the target is presented with no visual background [3, 33]. The illusions are consistent with altered proprioceptive input from the neck being used to judge the direction of gaze.

Electrical Stimulation

Electrical stimulation (ES) is a non-invasive technique [30] that provides nerve and/or muscle stimulation by means of surface electrodes. The characteristics, the size and the site of application of the electrodes and the characteristics of the electrical waves play a fundamental role in the neurophysiological effects of the ES. Usually, hand-held antalgic electro-stimulators are called TENS stimulators, which means transcutaneous electrical nerve stimulations [30]. The excitation of the peripheral motor nerves and the associated muscle activation is caused by the application of an electric current to the skin, usually correspond to the motor points. This kind of stimulation induces depolarization of the motor nerves either in the centrifugual or in the centripetal sense. Furthermore this kind of stimulation induces an activation of the sensitive nerves of the skin. Thus is difficult to divide the motor and the sensitive effects of the ES.

Our previous experimental experiences [1, 6-13] showed that vibration of the paravertebral muscles can be substituted by ES. Lackner [24] remarked that the vestibular nuclei are really polysensorial relays and that they are not only labyrinth correlated. The author underlined that it is not possible under natural circumstances to activate the vestibular receptors without implicating other force- sensitive receptor systems that convey information relevant to spatial orientation.

On the basis of this extensive, but physiologically justified, point of view of the vestibular system, we refer to superficial paravertebral electrical stimulation vestibular electro-stimulation (VES).

It was shown that neurophysiological effects of VES are strictly dependent on the characteristics of the electrical wave. Thus the definition of VES pertains only to those waves able to induce measurable neurophysiological cervico-spinal effects.

The Device

Either for experimentations or for clinical application we used an electro-stimulator, Agar. It is a small (25 x 36 x 91 mm) and light (88 g) portable device prepared at Hadassah University Hospital of Jerusalem (Israel) and approved by the the USA Food and Drug Administration (Fig. 1).

The mean currency intensity is 0.9 $\mu A/mm^2$ and the impulse currency intensity is 30 μA/mm², the maximum impluse power is 5 Watts and the maximum impulse charge is 22 μ Coulombs, the mean impulse charge is 0.55 Coulombs.

The device is able to produce different stimulation modes (Fig. 2):

Burst. This consists of short pulse series at a high frequency repeated at slow frequency. This stimulation mode is used for pain relief. The stimulation should be so strong that muscle contractions can be seen. Usually the electrode is placed on a large muscle near to the aching spot. Burst is not useful for vestibular stimulation.

TENS. It consists of short electric impulses and is used for pain relief. The stimulation must never be so strong that muscle contractions are found. The electrodes are normally placed on nerve paths leading away from the

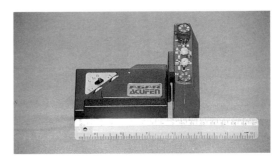

Fig. 1. The device

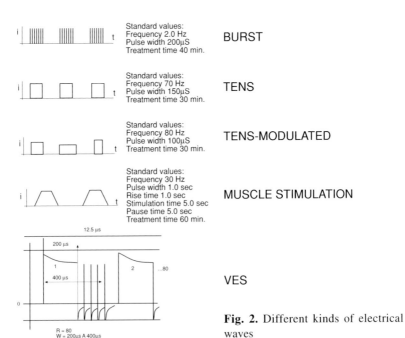

Fig. 2. Different kinds of electrical waves

aching spot. Sometimes this wave can be varied as regards both pulse width and stimulation currency. The variations are random but pulse width multiplied by stimulation current is constant (i.t = constant charge). This stimulation mode prevents tolerance to a set pulse width.

Muscle Stimulation Used for Rehabilitation of Muscles. The stimulation should be so strong that the muscles contract. The stimulation consists of stimulation (on time) with a slow rise (rise time) and a pause (off time). This sequence is repeated and makes the the muscle slowly contract and be tight for some time. It is often used on weak muscles (rehabilitation); the stimulation frequency is kept low (20-30 Hz) to avoid tiring out the muscle. For sports training higher frequencies are used. This wave is not useful for vestibular stimulation.

VES. This is a biphasic asymmetrical modulated square wave (Fig. 3). The modulation program randomly modifies the duration of each wave. The mean duration is 100 μs while the frequency is 80 Hz. Electrodes are small (2 cm square) and placed at a distance of 1 cm from each other. A pair of electrodes stimulates paravertebral muscles at the level of the second cervical vertebra, a pair stimulates the controlateral superior trapezius. The intensity of VES is never able to induce muscle contractions. The frequency used is in the muscle spindle range of vibratory activation (80 Hz). Thus, it is likely that VES activates the same spinal pathways of the CSRs. VES modulates the lower limbs postural reflexes in the same way.

Vibratory stimulation of muscle stimulation in a range between 1 and 100 Hz is able to activate muscle spindles [32]. The vibratory stimulation of the neck muscles produces proprioceptive inputs to the brainstem. These afferent volleys are able to evoke postural reflexes from the muscle of the lower limbs: CSRs. By means of the same mechanism, vibration is also able to evoke alterations of the perceptual reperesentation of the shape and orientation of the whole body and/or body parts.

The experimental results obtained by VES show that this kind of stimulation clearly influences the excitability of the motor neurons of the lower limbs. This influence resembled the action of CSRs on the extensor lower muscles.

Alteration of proprioceptive input from the neck by VES led to changed perception of head position. The manipulated proprioceptive input is incorporated in the head position signal with any other input contributing to head and body position control.

Indications

After whiplash injuries two conditions especially indicate for the VES treatment:

1. Paroxismal positional vertigo.
2. Unsteadyness and dizziness with VOR (vestibulo-ocular reflex) and/or VSR (vestibulo-spinal reflex) asymmetry.

Post-traumatic positional vertigo is, generally, atypical: it is often bilateral, not resolved by Semont manouvre. Nystagmus has no latency or it does not decrease by repeating the movements.

Usually we treat the patient with one or two Semont manouvres. When they are uneffective we employ VES. The electrodes are placed on the cervical paravertebral muscles ipsilateral to the fast phase of positioning nystagmus (that is usually concording with the vertiginous position) and on the contralateral trapezius. Each stimulation lasts 30 min. During stimulation the patient walks or performs simple and provocative rehabilitative exercises such as Cawthorn-Cooksey protocol. According to intensity of the symptoms the patient is treated once a day for 5 days a week for 2 weeks or once a day every 2 days for 2 weeks.

When paroxysmal positional vertigo is bilateral cervical electrodes are placed on the most intense side if there are no important VOR and/or VSR asymmetries.

When unsteadiness is associated with asymmetrical vestibular reflexes the cervical electrodes are placed on the opposite side of the VOR hyporeflexia and/or Romberg deviation and/or stepping deviation. In some cases VOR hyporeflexia is not accompanied by ipsilateral stepping and or Romberg deviation. This can be generally due either to the modification of the postural dynamic caused by the trauma or to pre-trauma postural conditions. In these cases it is sometimes difficult to interpret if VOR prevalence compensates VSR deficit, or if postural asymmetries compensate VOR hyporeflexia or if previous musculo-skeletal conditions induce unexpected VSRs. In these cases the sites of stimulation can not be standardized but have to be chosen on the basis of a complete postural evaluation and a complete neurootological examination with special regard to smooth pursuit, optokinetic nystagmus and VVOR (visuo-vestibulo-ocular reflex).

The general rule is that cervical electrodes are placed on the prevalent site and the trapezius electrodes are placed on the deficit site.

The treatment protocol lasts 2 weeks (a stimulation once a day) or 3 weeks (a stimulation every 2 days).

VES is frequently used to prepare the patient for reahabilitative treatment when vertigo and dizzines provoked by head/body is intense. There is no contraindication in the combination of VES and some early orthopedic treatment such as the collar. Obviously, in these cases VES is performed without the collar.

VES starting "equilibrium rehabilitation" in the early phases of the trauma and to treat also "low compliance" patients.

Some simple tasks during VES improve the effects of the treatment and the best results have been obtained combining VES and some cognitive involved rehabilitation procedures such as center of gravity visual feedback reeducation.

References

1. Alpini D, Cesarani A, Barozzi S (1992) Non pharmacological treatment of acute vertigo. In: Claussen CF, Kirtane MV, Schneider D (eds). Diagnostic procedures and imaging techniques used in neurotology. Proceedings of the XVI NES Congress, Dr Werner Rudat & Co, Nachf ed, m+p, Hamburg, pp 337-340
2. Berthoz A, Llinas R (1974) Afferent neck projection to the cat cerebellar cortex. Exp Brain Res 20:385-401
3. Biguer B, Donaldson IML, Hein A, Jannerod M (1988) Neck muscle vibration modifies the representation of visula motion and direction in man. Brain 111:1405-1424
4. Brink EE, Suzuki I, Timerick SJB, Wilson VJ (1985) Tonic neck reflex of the decerebrate cat: a role for propriospinal neurons. J Neurophysiol 54:978-987
5. Boyle R, Pompeiano O (1981) Convergence and interaction of neck and macular vestibular inputs on vestibulospinal neurons. J Neurophysiol 45:852-866
6. Cesarani A, Alpini D, Barozzi S (1990) Electrical stimulation in the treatment of acute vertigo. In: Sacristan T, Alvarez-Vincent JJ, Bartual J, Antoli-Candela F (eds). Otorhinolaryngology, head & neck surgery. Proceedings of the XIV World Congress of Otorhinolaryngology, Madrid, 1989, Kugler & Ghedini Publ, Amsterdam, Berkeley, Milano
7. Cesarani A, Alpini D, Barozzi S (1990) Neck electrical stimulation in the treatment of labyrinth acute vertigo. Riv It EEG Neurof Cl 13(1): 55-61
8. Cesarani A, Pertoni T, Alpini D (1988) L'electrostimulation cervicale posteriore dans la rehabilitation des handicaps vestibulaires. XXII Reunion de la Societe d'Otoneurologie de Langue Francaise, Toulose, May
9. Cesarani A, Alpini D, Barozzi S (1989) L'electrostimulation electrique dans la reeducation vestibulaire: indications, limites, perspectives. XXIII Reunion de la Societe d'Otoneurologie de Langue Francaise, Modena, June
10. Cesarani A, Alpini D (1991) New trends in rehabilitation treatment of vertigo and dizziness. In: Akyildiz N, Portmann M (eds). Vertigo and its treatment. Proceedings of International Symposium for Prof G Portmann's Centenary, Ankara, 16-18 Maggio 1990, pp 90-104
11. Cesarani A, Alpini D, Barozzi S (1992) Superficial paravertebral electrical stimulation. A conservative treatment of vertigo and dizziness. In: Claussen CF, Kirtane MV, Schneider D (eds). Conservative versus surgical treatment of sensorineural hearing loss, tinnitus, vertigo and nausea. Proceedings of the XVIII NES Congress, Dr Werner Rudat & Co, Nach. edi, m+p, Hamburg
12. Cesarani A, Alpini D, Barozzi S, Osio M (1993) Superficial paravertebral electrical stimulation (SPES) in the treatment of vertigo and disequilibrium disturbances. In: Dufour A (ed). Proceedings XXVII symposium Societe d'Oto-Neurologie de Langue Francaise Sanremo, p 47

13. Cesarani A (1994) The cervical electrostimulation. Neurootology Newsletter 1(1):67-72
14. Corbin KB, Hinsey JC (1935) Intramedullary course of the dorsal root fibers of each of the first four cervical nerves. J Comp Meurol 63:119-126
15. Frederickson JM, Schwarz D, Kornhuber HH (1966) Convergence and interaction of vetsibular and deep somatic afferents upon neurons in the vestibular nuclei of the cat. Acta Otolaryngol, Stoch, 61:168-188
16. Fukuda T (1961) Studies on human dynamic postures from the viewpoint of postural reflexes. Acta Oto-Laryngol [Suppl 161]:1-52
17. Ghez C (1991) Posture. In: Kandel ER, Schwartz JH, Jessel TM (eds). Principles of neural science. 3rd ed, Elsevier, New York, 596-607
18. Hagbart KE (1973) The effect of muscle vibration in normal man and in patients with motor disordersin. In: Desmedt JE (ed). New developments in electromyography and clinical neurophysiology. Karger AG, Basel, 3:428-443
19. Hikosaka O, Maeda M (1973) Cervical effects on abducens motoneurons and their interaction with vestibulo-ocular reflex. Exp Brain Res 18:512-530
20. Igarashi M, Alford BR, Watanabe T, Maxiam PM (1969) Role of the neck proprioceptors for the maintenance of dynamic bodily equilibrium in the squirrel momkey. Laryngoscope 79:1713-1727
21. Karnath HO, Christ K, Hartjie W (1993) Decrease of controlateral neglect by neck muscle vibration and spatial orientation of the trunk midline. Brain 116:383-396
22. Kobayashi Y, Toshiaki, Kamio T (1988) The role of cervical inputs in compensation for unilateral labyrinthectomized patients. Adv Oto-Rhino-Laryng 42:185-189
23. Lackner JR (1988) Some proprioceptive influences on the perceptual representation of body shape and orientation. Brain 111:281-297
24. Lackner JR (1992) Multimodal and motor influences on orientatiom: implications for adapting to weightless and virtual environments. J Vest Res 2:307-322
25. Lindasy KW, Roberts TDM, Rosemberg JR (1976) Asymmetric tonic labyrinth refelexes and their interaction with neck reflexes in the decerebrate cat. J Physiol, London, 261:583-601
26. MacClosey DI (1973) Differences between the senses of movement and position shown by the effects of loading and vibration of muscles in man. Brain Research, Amsterdam, 61:119-131
27. Manzoni D, Pompeiano O, Stampacchia G (1979) Tonic cervical influences on posture and reflex movements. Arch Ital Biol 117:81-110
28. Maeda M (1979) Neck influences on the vestibulo-ocular reflex arc and the vestibulo-cerebellum. Prog Brain Res 50:551-559
29. Mergner T, Anastasopoulos K, Becjer W, Deecke L (1981) Comparison of the modes of interaction of labyrinthine and neck afferents in the suprasylvian cortex and vestibular nuclei of the cat. Progress in oculomotor research. Fuchs and Becker (eds). Elsevier, 343-350
30. Poumarat G (1993) Les electrostimulateurs. Cah Kinesither 164(6):3-13
31. Raymond J, Sans A (1979) Projections somato-sensorielles dans les noyaux vestibulaires. Etude Electrphysiologique. J Physiol, Paris, 75:269-274
32. Roll JP, Rol R (1991) From eye to foot: a proprioceptive chain involved in postural control. In: Cesarani A, Alpini D (eds). Diagnosi e trattamento dei disturbi

dell'equilibrio nell'età evolutiva e involutiva. B e G Editori, Verona, 93-104

33. Tokinaze T, Murao M, Ogata T, Kondo T (1951) Electromyographic studies on tonic neck, lumbar, and labyrinthine reflexes in normal persons. Jap J Physiol 2:130-146

34. Wilson VJ, Maeda M, Franck JI (1975) Input from neck afferent to the cat flocculus. Brain Res 89:133-138

Neurophysiological Investigation of the Relation Between Vestibular Activation and Cervicospinal Reflex

M. Osio, L. Brunati[1], G. Abello[2] and A. Mangoni

Bending the neck and turning the head respecting to the body cause the stimulation of the cervical proprioceptors. This kind of receptors activate a pathway projecting to the vestibular nuclei.

The impulses are reflected through the nucleo-reticular formation and then to the spinal cord. Such activation allows movements of the neck to influence the postural set and to modify the activation of the antigravitary muscles of the lower limbs (Fig. 1).

This pattern of muscolar activation is hypotized on the basis of the so-called neck-postural reflexes, or better named cervico-spinal reflex [1]. During the contraction of the paravertebral muscles of the neck there is a response characterized by inhibition of ispilateral soleus respect to the side of neck stimulation and facilitation of the controlateral muscles [2]. During the superficial electrical stimulation (SES) the paraspinal muscles are also activated and there are previous studies that show that SES is able to reduce vertigo and dizziness [3]. This kind of stimulation is also able to evoke changes in activity of the muscles of the legs. We used a neurophysiological test named H-reflex to control this modification. It holds special interest because it can attest the activation of the vestibular-spinal way during the stimulation of the paraspinal muscles through the modification of exitability of the motoneuron. Under appropriate conditions, a single electrical shock to the tibial nerve will evoke two discrete motor action potentials in the calf muscles. The first potential, the M-wave, result from direct stimulation of motor nerve fibers. The second potential, the H-wave, is the expression of a monosynaptic reflex, which runs in afferent fibers (II a) from the neuromuscolar spindles and back again through motor afferents.

Since no interneurons are involved, the size of the second action potential will provide a measure of motoneuron excitability under a variety of experimental conditions [4]. Eight normal subjects (5 females and 3 males), aged between 20-33 years old, were admitted to the study.

———

Clinica Neurologica, I Università di Milano, Italy
[1] Fondazione Pro Juventute, Don Carlo Gnocchi, Milan, Italy
[2] Fondazione Pro Juventute, Don Carlo Gnocchi, Politecnico di Milano, Italy

Labyrynthic Receptors

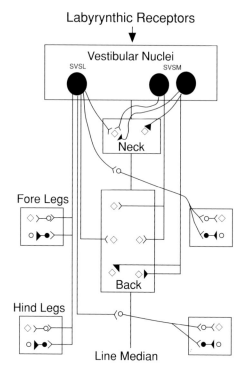

Fig. 1. Connections between vestibular nuclei and limbs motoneurons in the cat

Subject did all sit in a comfortable armchair, with cervical spine at rest position with non flexion, extension or lateral bending and head support and not rotated with respect the trunk.

Legs were at rest and supported, the hips were flexed at 90°, the knee were flexed at 120° and the ankles were flexed at 90°. Patients were in a quiet room, were awake and relaxed with eyes closed.

Recording of the H-Reflex were obtained with pregelled surface electrodes. Active electrode was fixed on the distal on the belly of soleous muscle, while references electrode was fixed 30 mm below. Stimulation of the tibial nerve was performed with surface electrodes at the popliteal fossa. Interelectrodes distance was 25 mm. Stimulus duration was 1 ms. All this in accordance with the indication of the literature [5]. Stimulus intensity was between 5 and 21 mA at the intensity need to evoke the maximum amplitude of the H-Reflex (H Max) for each subject.

H Max from soleous muscle right and left legs were recorded every five minutes before, during and after the stimulation of the muscles. In particular superficial electrical stimulation (SES) of neck paravertebral muscles and contemporary controlateral upper part of the trapezius was applied. SES of the neck muscles was applied with pulse rate of 80 Hz and a pulse width randomly modulated between 100-200 μs of duration. First SES application was performed for 15 min contemporaneously on the right paravertebral muscles of the neck and on the left upper part of trapezius muscle. After 30 minutes SES was applied to the controlateral paravertebral of the neck and trapezius muscle for a duration of 15 minutes. The recordings of the H Max were obtained by left and right leg. We calculated mean (M) and Standard Deviation (SD) of the 5 consecutive H Max responses and obtained value were tabulated. Measures of H Max value were done every 5 min. In this way, for each subject were recorded one H Max basal value before application SES, 3 H Max were obtained every five minutes during SES applied to the right paravertebral and left trapezius muscle; 3-6 H Max during to recovery phase, one H Max basal, 3 H Max values during SES applied to the left paravertebral muscle and right trapezius muscle and 3-6 H Max values obtained during a second recovery phase. Statistical analysis was performed with the Student's t test comparing H Max recorded before, during and after each SES application.

Results were homogeneous in all subjects both for the stimulation patterns.

The contemporary SES of the left paravertebral cervical muscles and of the right trapezius enhanced in all subjects after 10 min, H Max amplitude (14% of the maximum amplitude; $p = 0.02$) of the right soleous muscle and reduced, after 15 minutes, H Max amplitude (- 20%; $p = 0.001$) of the soleous muscles. H Max amplitude returned to the basal values 10 minutes after the end of the stimulation on the right soleous and was still reduced (- 36%; $p = 0.001$) 10 minutes after the end of SES on the left soleous. In some subjects H Max values lasted less than normal for 30 minutes after the end of SES. Recording from the right soleous showed that 10 minutes after the end of SES amplitude was still decreased (27%; $p = 0.001$) in some subject inhibition of the H reflex lasted over 30 minutes (Fig. 2).

The stimulation by SES of the right paravertebral cervical muscles and left trapezius induced, after 5 minutes, an increase of the left side values (20%; $p = 0.001$) and reduced, after 15 minutes, the amplitude of the right values (- 32%; $p = 0.001$). In a short time after the end of the SES left H reflex returns to basal values. Then a paradoxal second phase begins H reflex decreases slowly but progressively reaching a new "basal" value that is significatively ($p = 0.001$) lower. Right H reflex remains reduced at least 10 minutes after the end of SES (- 27%; $p = 0.001$) (Fig. 3).

The results of the present study showed that SES of the neck muscles clearly influenced the excitability of the motor neurons of the lower limbs.

It is important to underline that SES at the intensity to which was applied never evoked muscles contraction. On the contrary SES was applied in the same frequency range (80 Hz) which is able to activate muscles spindles by vibratory stimulation. Thus, it is likely that SES activate the same spinal pathways activated from the cervicospinal reflexes, modulating in the same

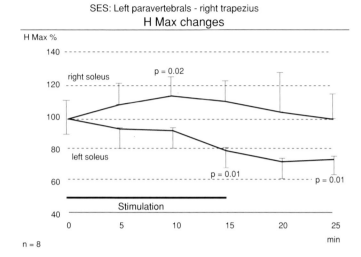

Fig. 2. Effects of electrical stimulation on H-reflexes

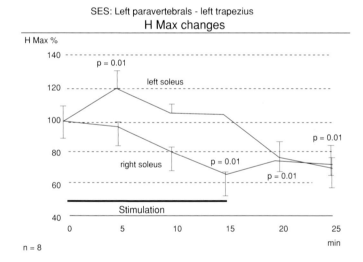

Fig. 3. Effects of electrical stimulation on H-reflexes

way the postural reflexes of the lower limbs. This action is probably mediated from proprioceptive input originated in the spindles of the neck muscles. Otherwise we can not exclude the action of skin receptors mediating the vibratory sense.

Proprioceptive afferent input evoked from SES of the neck muscles could reach also controlateral Deiters vestibular nuclei and cortex, probably by mean of reticular pathways. In such way SES may influence the equilibrium system. It is know [1] that if vestibular apparatus is damaged, the reflexes of the neck, limb and eyes muscles become preminent.

Therefore it is possible that SES action in treatment of vertigo and dizziness is based on the modulation of the proprioceptive input from neck muscles.

At last there is the observation that inhibitory effect is more pronounced and long lasting than the excitatory one. Supraspinal pathway activation may give account of this phenomena but further investigations are needed to verify such hypothesis.

References

1. Ghez C (1991) Posture. In: Kaendel ER, Schwartz JH, Jessell TM (eds). Principles of Neural Sciences. 3rd Ed, Elsevier, New York, Amsterdam, London, Tokyo, 596-607
2. Ghelarducci B (1994) Funzioni vestibolari ed organizzazione globale del movimento. Riabilitazione Oggi, XI, 6:15-21
3. Alpini D, Cesarani A, Barozzi S (1992) Non pharmacological treatment of acute vertigo. In: Claussen CF, Wirtane MV, Schneider D (eds). Diagnostic Procedures and Imagining Techniques used in Neurotology. Proceedings of the XVI NES CONGRESS. Werner Rudat & Co, Nachf ed m + p, Hambourg 337-340
4. Angel RW, Hofmann WW (1963) The H Reflex in Normal, Spastic and Rigid Subjects. Archives of Neurology, Vol 8, June, 21-26
5. Kots Ya M (1979) The Organization of Voluntary Movement. Neurophysiological Mechanisms. Plenum Press, New York, London, II, 27-50

The Therapeutic Strategy

A. CESARANI AND D. ALPINI[1]

Introduction

Training focused on the primary functional problems and secondary adaptive strategies of the individual can have positive effects on postural stability in post-whiplash vertigo and dizziness. The most effective training program, however, incorporates all the information from the patient's history, physical examination, clinical and instrumental test results.

The Equilibrium system has to be considered, in a cybernetic point of view, as a complex open system. It is complex because it is comprised of different sub-systems interconnected in a way by which the functional effect of the system is different and more complex than the mere sum of each sub-system effects. It is open because it is interconnected with the enviroment, too, and it is modifiable by the environment itself [17].

Cybernetics of the Equilibrium System

A system is defined as any set of variables that the experimenter selects among those available in the real machine.

A variable is defined as a measurable quantity which at every instant has a numerical value (e.g. pressure,temperature, angle, electrical potentials) [1-3]. A system can be also defined as a collection of components arranged and interconnected in a definite way: a system is any collection of communicating materials and processes which together perform some function.

By this point of view labyrinths, eyes, vestibular nuclei, paravertebral proprioceptors, antigravity extensor muscles of the lower limbs and spine, ocularmotor muscles and plantar receptors constitute a system, the equilibrium system.

Ospedale Maggiore Policlinico, Istituto di Audiologia, Università degli Studi di Milano, Via Sforza 35, Milan, Italy
[1] ENT, Otoneurological Service Scientific Institute S. Maria N.te, F.ne don Gnocchi, Via Capecelatro 66 - 20148 Milan, Italy

Systems are generally grouped into five main categories regarding their different cybernetic aspects [2]:

1. Lumped systems: the physical dimensions of the elements which constitute it are very small compared to the wave length of the input-output quantitaties. The system is "distributed".
2. Time invariant systems and time varying systems: the system is time invariant if the elements of the system do not change their values with time, otherwise the system is time varying.
3. Linear systems: these must meet the homogeneity and superposition criteria and the operators for input-output relation are independent of both input and output quantities. Other systems are "nonlinear".
4. Causal systems: a system which does not give any output unless an excitation is applied to its input is so defined. Otherwise a system is "uncausal". If an uncausal system is, in addition, free, linear and time invariant, it is called "autonomous".
5. Passive systems: in such systems all the elements are passive. If there are dependent or independent active elements or energy sources, the system is active.

The behaviour of any system is determined by [4]:

- The characteristics of the components or subsystems (e.g. threshold of stimulation of γ-motoneurons, or characteristics of endolymph).
- The structure of communication between components, which usually involves feedback paths (e.g. internuclear vestibular connections, cerebello-vestibular inhibitory pathways).
- The input signals or variables to the systems initially assumed to be independent variables under the investigator's control.

The results of the system's operation upon the inputs are the outputs. Any variable of the system may be considered an output.

Synergetics of the Equilibrium System

The human brain is, maybe, the most complex system in the universe. Its several hundred billion elements, organized at various levels of description, permit the organism to interact adaptively with a wide variety of enviroments. The brain perceives sudden serial and intermodal integrated inner and outer stimuli and it programs coordinate reactions (physical and/or psychical). With this point of view the human brain may be considered a site of reactions rather than a site of action. Perception ability is, in fact, the functional basis of movement learning and it is sometimes more important than motor production skill. This is true especially for that particular motor skill named "equilibrium".

Equilibrium is a complex system that provides two main functions: (1)

coordination and (2) orientation.

The main function *coordination* (EA) is subdivided into three main sub-functions:

EAa: Coordination of eye movement with head and body movement with respect to continuous, dinstinct, foveal vision.

EAb: Coordination of tonic antigravity muscle contraction and gravity force in order to maintain the desired position and shape of the body (so-called posture).

EAc: Coordination of tonic muscle contraction with gravity force and with dynamic phasic muscle contraction in order to obtain the desired movement (walking, stepping, running, jumping) into the environment.

The main function *orientation* (EB) is subdivided into two main subfunctions:

EBa: Perception of the orientation of each part of the body with respect to each other part (perception of the body shape) [19].

EBb: Perception of the orientation of the whole body with respect to the environment.

Simplifing we can state that coordination subfunctions concern "outself" representation while orientation subfunctions concern "itself" representation.

A model system approach that currently holds considerable promise for understanding of the higher level processes of internal both itself and outself representation is the study of spatial behaviour. Spatial orientation involves the integration of complex, polysensory information and associative memory both for complex stimulus configurations and for the conditional consequences of the organism's own movement with respect to the sources of these stimuli.

Finally, spatial cognition requires the computation, either from previous experience or from relatively "hardwired" circuitry, of spatially equivalent sequences of movements leading to the generation of novel trajectories between various starting locations and some goal.

The brain uses repetitive sampling to analyze the complex stimuli with which it is confronted. Although collecting successive samples of stimuli and extracting different information from them may be a routine operation, the machinery involved must be complex indeed, involving interaction and synchronization of activities in sensory and motor systems.

The aim of the complex open equilibrium system is arranged in different subsystems, interconnected with the enviroment by means of different sensorial subsystems (inputs): (a) labyrinthic; (b) visual; (c) proprioceptive (from spine joints, paravertebral muscles and antigravity lower limbs muscles); (d) somatoesthesic (especially from the feet).

The inputs are integrated in vestibular nuclei, reticular formation and cerebellum. These integrations are controlled by the cortex.

The output motor subsystems are aimed at coordinating eye-head movement (balance ocular-motor reflexes) and to maintain equilibrium during standing or walking (balance spinal reflexes).

Functional characteristics of the equilibrium system are the same as the complex open systems in general and its rules are the same as those of the complex open systems; knowledge of these rule is the corner-stone of therapeutic strategy for every kind and site of lesion. The equilibrium system is ruled by the following laws [1, 5-7]:

TOTALITY: Every component of the system correlates with the other components. In this way a modification of one component has effects on the other parts and on the whole system. In the equilibrium system a modification of the proprioceptive inputs may modify the vestibulo-ocular reflex; modification of the center of gravity (CoG) may modify the activity of antigravity lower limb muscles.

FEEDBACK: Every open system is a circular system in which the outputs of the system are inputs themselves. In the equilibrium system the outputs are muscle reflexes. Muscle activity is itself a proprioceptive input to the system.

EQUIFINALITY: In a circular self-regulated system the same functional effect can be obtained by means of action of different components or different arrangements of system components. This is the cybernetic basis for sensory substitution during compensation of vestibular lesions. Balance is maintained using diferent sensorimotor strategies in different persons and/or in different conditions. The same (equifinality) balance results are obtained either in normal subjects or in compensated vestibular neuritis patients when the interrelations between the different components of the system have been modified.

CALIBRATION: A system is steady if the components of the system remain within defined limits. This is the cybernetic explanation of symptomatology threshold that may be different in different patients.

PREFERENCE: Each equilibrium system is preferentially arranged in a precise and "personal" sensorimotor organization. Each subject maintains his antigravity position using preferentially visual, vestibular, proprioceptive or somatoesthesic inputs.

REDUNDANCE: The equilibrium system is based on redundant sensorial (sensory redundance) inputs and redundant motor programs (motor redundance) [8, 9].

The Role of Brainstem and Cerebellum

Cerebellum and brainstem circuits are essential for the development and expression of the most basic form of associative learning. Normal human movements performed under an equilibrium condition, can be considered to be harmonic with a continuous interconnection of coordination and orientation. These interconnected "movements", in each instant, are based also on psychological and and attentive subject mental sets (so-called cognitive aspects of equilibrium) and they are regulated on the basis of visual, vestibular, auditory and proprioceptive feedbacks [12].

If we consider normal human equilibrium as the result of an accumulated interactive, associative and unconscious *learning*, we also can interpretate equilibrium disorders as the results of disadaptative, unassociative, sensorimotor uncoordinated and unfinalized movements. Nystagmus itself has to be considered a disadaptative and not finalized movement of the eyes. One of the most important functions of the whole brain and, especially, of the cerebellum is, in fact, the ability to inhibit uncoordinated and unfinalized motor activities and, contemporarily, to facilitate those functions that allow human physical and psychical perceiving. The selective ability of unuseful activities inhibition and useful activities facilitation is one of the functional bases of the "plasticity" of the brain.

The two principal inputs to the cerebellum are climbing and mossy fibers. Climbing fibers come entirely from the neurons of a structure in the brain stem termed the inferior olive. The climbing fibers send collaterals to the deep nuclei and project to the cerebellar cortex, where a given Purkinje cell receives a powerful excitatory synaptic input from one, and only one, climbing fiber.

The inferior olive receives its primary sensory input from the somatic sensory systems (skin, joints, pain) but it is also connected to other sensory circuits.

The mossy fibers originate predominantly from neurons in the pontine nuclei of the brainstem, but from other sources as well, for example, direct somatic sensory input. They project to the cerebellar cortex, where they synapse on granule cells. Mossy fibers also send collaterals to the deep nuclei.

The granule cells project to the Purkinje cells as parallel fibers. A given parallel fiber contacts hundreds of Purkinje cells with excitatory synapses. The pontine nuclei receive projections from many places in the brain, including important projections from the cerebral cortex. In terms of input to the cerebellar cortex, the climbing and mossy-parallel fiber systems are thus quite differently organized. The responses of a Purkinje cell to mossy-parallel fiber activation and climbing fiber activation are quite different. Thus, the activation by parallel fibers yields single action potentials, termed "simple spikes". The spontaneous rate of activation of Purkinje cells by granule cells (parallel fibers) is quite variable and can range as high 50/s or more. Activation of a Purkinje cell by a climbing fiber yields a very brief, train of action potentials (several hundreds per second) that lasts for only a few spikes. This Purkinje cell response to activation by a climbing fiber is termed "complex spike". The simple spike response to parallel fiber activation and the complex spike response to climbing fiber activation are easily distinguished in extracellular single unit recording from a Purkinje cell.

There are several types of inhibitory interneurons in cerebellar cortex such as Golgi cells, stellate cells, and basket cells. Indeed the only excitatory neurons in cerebellar cortex are the granule cells giving rise to the parallel fibers. All other neurons in cerebellar cortex are inhibitory and are thought to use γ-amino-butyric acid (GABA) as their inhibitory neurotransmitter. The Golgi neurons are activated primarily by parallel fibers that then make inhibitory synapses on granule cells, thereby constituting an inhibitory feedback loop. The stellate and basket cells are activated by the parallel fibers and exert inhibition on the Purkinje cells (feed-forward inhibition).

The only output from the cerebellum comes from the cerebellar deep nuclei which project both to higher brain structures and to lower brain structures (interpositus). Purkinje cells are the only neurons that project information out from the cerebellar cortex and they project only to the deep nuclei. Furthermore, their synaptic actions are thought to be entirely inhibitory.

Like the cerebral cortex, there are several different regions of cerebellar cortex that contain representations or maps of the body; information about events of the skin of the body are represented in multiple redundance. But unlike those in cerebral cortex, these maps do not have topological "coherence". In cerebellar cortex the representation of various regions of the body appear to be chaotic (e.g. eyelid region next to finger one). This incoherent mapping has been termed "fractured somatotopy".

The climbing fibers have very localized and powerfully excitatory actions on Purkinje cells. This organization led theorists to the notion that the localized climbing fiber input acts on cerebellar cortex as the *teaching* input while the distributed mossy-parallel fiber input acts as the *learning* input.

Mutatis mutandis, with classical theoretical and modern computational models we can attribute to cerebellum a main role in *motor learning* and in *equilibrium teaching* [13].

The main functional differences between equilibrium disorders in cerebellum injuries versus brainstem injuries are essentially based on these distinctions:

- Brainstem contributes to movement and equilibrium informing the cerebellum and providing to the cerebellum *learning* information.
- Cerebellum learns through sensorial and proprioceptive feedback (via the brainstem) and *teaches* the brainstem how it has to learn, regulating, in this way, movements and equilibrium.

An experimental set aimed to evaluate the role of the cerebellum in motor (and equilibrium) "teaching" is the evaluation of adaptative behaviour of the vestibulo-ocular-reflex (VOR) to the changing conditions brought about naturally, by cell loss, disease, and aging, or artificially in the laboratory, by prism glasses that alter the visual field.

The ability of the cerebellum to detect and repair this "dysmetria" that would otherwise cause motor incoordination indicates that more than a simple open loop control system is involved; feedback as to the accuracy of the eye movements is clearly being provided to the cerebellum by the visual system. Thus a slip of the retinal image signals the cerebellum to recalibrate the VOR. This recalibration signal must indicate the exact nature of the necessary change in the VOR, for example, how much of an increase or decrease in the gain will correctly recalibrate the reflex.

According to Robinson [18] vestibulocerebellum is the main instigator of VOR adaptative behaviour. Robinson defined the vestibulocerebellum as the "flocculi, the ventral paraflocculi, the lateral third of dorsal paraflocculi, the nodulus, the uvula, the lower half of lobe VIII, and the lower three or four lobules of the paramedian lobules". The author found the vestibulocerebellum to be critical in the maintenance of the VOR. After vestibulocerebellar lesions, the VOR remained unchangeable no matter what was done. Robinson's work indicates that the vestibulocerebellum is necessary to produce and maintain the large plastic changes that are observed in the VOR when it must adapt to changes in visual field.

Subsequent works by Ito [14, 15] further established that the flocculus region of the vestibulocerebellum is critical for adaptation. The primary vestibular fibers project to the flocculus as mossy fibers. The flocculus also receives climbing fibers from the retina that, according to Ito, contain error information about retinal slip: the discrepancy between the image that ought to project to the fovea and the "erroneous" image that does project to the fovea. It should be noted that the precise locus or loci of neuronal plasticity that code adaptation of the VOR is still a matter of discussion, but authors agree that the cerebellar cortex of the flocculus is necessary for adaptation of the VOR and there is experimental evidence of memory trace location either in cerebellar cortex or in interpositus nucleus. The medial vestibular nucleus participates in cerebellum control of VOR adaptation and,in fact, it can be considered a deep cerebellar nucleus, displaced to the brainstem, in terms of its connections, for example, monosynaptic projection of Purkinje cell axons.

Fujita [10, 11] proposed an "adaptative filter" model of the cerebellum to formally account for the adaptive abilities of the VOR. While modulating the VOR, Purkinje cells are presumed to receive sinusoidal input of various phases from the mossy fibers via the granule cells and parallel fibers. Within this model the Purkinje cells learn to respond selectively to the various phase version until they only respond to a very specific combination of inputs; that is to say, they adjust the synaptic weights on the parallel fiber inputs so that, when summed at the Purkinje cell, the desired output is produced. In Fujita's adaptive filter model, Purkinje cells are presumed to perform a filtering function on the basis of multiple pairs of input signals and corresponding desired output signals. The Golgi cells are postulated to work as phase lag elements that act as leaky integrators with a time constant of a few seconds. The output from this network, that is, the parallel fiber signals, would then reperesent different versions of compensators at different phase lags, depending on the relative weights of the inputs. The outputs of the parallel fiber signals are gathered together through various synaptic connenctions, which possess modifiable weights, to form the desired Purkinje cell output, that is, the final signal. The weights assigned to the individual parallel fiber signals are adaptive and plastic. They are adjustable depending on the desired output and how close the actual output of the Purkinje cells is to this desired output. The climbing fiber afferent inputs into the cerebellum which originate in the inferior olive and form powerful excitatory synapses with the Purkinje cells are presumed [10, 11, 16] to be responsible for the *learning* capabilities of the adaptive filter. In other words, the mossy fiber afferent carry information to be processed by the cerebellum and the climbing fiber afferents carry *teaching* signals to the Purkinje cells.The activity of the climbing filter inputs is determined by the discrepancy between the actual and the desired Purkinje cell output relative to its spontaneous discharge rate.

A close parallel can be drawn between the error signaling role of the climbing fibers in adaptation of the VOR and the reinforcing or teaching role of the climbing fibers in classical conditioning pavlovian experiments.

Two quite different behavioural forms of learning, classical conditioning of discrete behavioural responsens and adaptation of the VOR have converged quite remarkably toward a common neural substrate. The cerebellum and its associated brainstem circuitry are necessary and sufficient for both forms of behavioural plasticity. In both paradigms a key event is a depression in the frequency of firing of Purkinje cells as a result of training or adaptation. A decrease in Purkinje cell firing will yield an increased neuronal response in interpositus (classical conditioning) or in vestibular nuclei (VOR adaptation), which increases the probability of a behaviour response [14].

The characteristics of equilibrium disorders in brainstem and/or cerebellum diseases and their treatment possibilities depend on the different interactions between learning and teaching. In other words, we can state that brainstem teaches the cerebellum to learn what the cerebellum itself has to teach to brainstem itself, that is to say, that in brainstem inputs and ouputs run parallel while in cerebellum these two signals cross and interconnect and a large disruption can be caused by small lesions.

Treatment possibilities are entirely based on the residual capability of brainstem *learning* and cerebellum *teaching*.

According to this kind of model it is easy to understand that the dysfunction will be as worse and the treatment possibilities will be as reduced if the injury regards the teacher (cerebellum) while therapeutic results will be potentially better if the injury regards the learner (brainstem).

The Therapeutic Strategy

Planning of the treatment of equilibrium disorders in a patient affected with equilibrium disturbances requires answering two main questions:
1. Is the dysfunctional system again under the control of the fundamental laws totality and equifinality?
2. Is the center able again to integrate sensorial inputs comparing differrent sensorimotor patterns?

On the basis of the answers to these questions two general conditions may be considered: (1) The complex equilibrium system is again ruled by the laws. Equilibrium disorders are mainly caused by a "quantitative" decreasing of the sensorial inputs, or motor outputs, or central integration of sensorimotor patterns. (2) The system is no longer ruled by the laws of normal complex open systems. Equilibrium disorders are mainly caused by a "qualitative" decreasing of central sensorimotor integration.

The treatment of disorders grouped in the first condition is mainly based on neurorehabilitation. The sytem is, in fact, a "legal" system in which the therapist can act on the basis of the laws of totality, equifinality, feedback, calibration, redundance. On the basis of vestibular responses excitatory (nicergoline, gingko biloba, piracetam) or inhibitory drugs (cinarrizine, flunarizine) may be employed, too. On the basis of general vascular conditions some pathogenetic (aspirine, ticlopidine) drugs are associated.

In these patients neurorehabilitation increases the activity of good peripheral inputs acting on sensorial and motor redondance. Prognostic evaluation is based on three specific goals: (1) the primary damage: the structural lesion of one or more equilibrium subsystem; (2) the secondary damage: functional imbalance of sub-systems not directly involved by the lesion such as equilibrium disorders caused by post-lesional postural syndromes; (3) the tertiary damage: the crystalization of pathological sensorimotor patterns and/or psychological avoiding behaviours.

Rehabilitation is likely pointed toward limiting the primary damage, reducing the secondary damage, avoiding the tertiary damage.

Rehabilitation is based either on peripheral sensorial and motor redundance or on central spontaneous compensation mechanisms: functional sensorial substitution, structural reorganization, recalibration of sensorimotor patterns, internuclear inhibition). Drugs are given to increase neural plasticity by means of axonal sprouting and reorganization of neural networks,

Weakness of ankle joint muscles, loss of ankle sensation, reduced mobility of the ankles are contraindications for movement strategy training unless the underlying physiologic factors are also addressed.

Contraindications to teaching appropriate use of hip movements might include weakness or loss of mobility about the hip joints. There is also clinical evidence suggesting that patients with profound loss of peripheral vestibular function cannot effectively coordinate hip movements and that training in these cases is ineffective.

The treatment of disorders grouped in the second condition is mainly based on drugs. This system is, in fact, an "illegal" system in which the therapist cannot act on the basis of cybernetic laws. Drugs are employed with the aim of regaining a circular, cybernetic system in which a correct sub-system interconnection allows rehabilitation. The different behaviour of the legal and illegal equilibrium pathological systems is caused by: the pre-lesional characteristics of the patient; the quantitative characteristics of the lesion; the qualitative characteristics of the disease; and the side of lesion/s.

The side of the lesion induces different therapeutic strategies.

Clinical Cases

Case number 1 - Acute

The patient is a 24 year old healthy woman. Whiplash injury occurred on December 20th. It was examined for the first time on December 22nd. She complained of cervical stiffness and pain, vertigo provoked by head and body movements and unsteadiness. No fractures were documented at X-ray. No neurological symptoms were present. No significant VOR asymmetries were revealed at ENG. Saccades were normal, smooth pursuit and optokinetic gains were slightly reduced at 40°/s (0.65 for smooth pursuit and 0.6 for OKN).

Figure 1 compares cranio-corpography performed with (A) and without (B) collar. In both cases no significant deviations were revealed but the pattern shows cervico-cephalic incoordination especially without a collar.

Figure 2 shows stabilometric results without a collar and Fig. 3 with a collar: body sway with closed eyes is significantly improved by the collar.

On the basis of neuro-otologic findings the patient used a cervical collar for 15 days together with myorelaxants and antiflammatory drugs. No particular rehabilitative treatment was planned.

After 2 weeks cranio-corpography without a collar confirmed (Fig. 4) cervico-cephalic incoordination, and stabilometry without collar confirmed pathological body sway with eyes closed.

A physical and instrumental rehabilitative treatment was planned for 2 weeks (one treatment a day for 5 days a week and simplest Cawthorn-Cooksey exercises once a day, every day):
1. Balance coordination exercises with eyes closed on soft mattress.
2. Balance on one leg either with visual feed-back or with eyes closed.
3. Mobilization of dorso-lumbar spine.
4. Stretching of cervical muscles and trapezius.

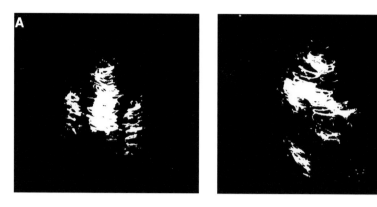

Fig. 1 A, B. Craniocorpography with (**A**) and without (**B**) collar

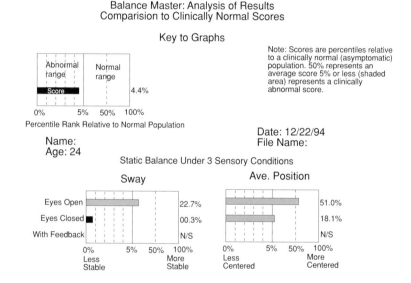

Balance Master: Analysis of Results
Comparision to Clinically Normal Scores

Key to Graphs

Note: Scores are percentiles relative to a clinically normal (asymptomatic) population. 50% represents an average score 5% or less (shaded area) represents a clinically abnormal score.

Percentile Rank Relative to Normal Population

Name:
Age: 24

Date: 12/22/94
File Name:

Static Balance Under 3 Sensory Conditions

Sway

Ave. Position

Fig. 2. Stabilometric results without collar

5. Isometric retropositioning of the head during pelvic mobilization either in charging or discharging positions.
6. Sequences of motor coordinated steps first with eyes open, then with eyes closed.
7. Skitter exercises: forward leg extensions; backward leg extensions; ankle-hip strategies; oscillations; slalom.
8. Exercises 1-2-3-8 (especially 8A and 8E) performed using vestibular electrical stimulation (VES).

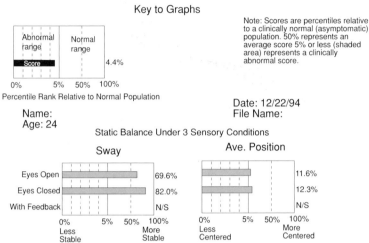

Fig. 3. Stabilometric results with collar

After rehabilitation the patient continued some exercises of the Cawthorne-Cooksey protocol at home. Figures 5 and 6 show cranio-corpographic and stabilometric findings 3 months after whiplash: balance is normal.

Case number 2 - Chronic

The patient is a 70 year old man. Whiplash injury occurred 3 years before. After the accident he complained of worsening of previous left hypoacusis until anacusis, slight worsening of right medium hypoacusis, acute vertigo attacks lasting some hours, position vertigo and subcontinuous unsteadiness. After 3 years the vertigo attacks were gone but dysequilibrium was important.

Saccades showed increased delay and reduced accuracy, smooth pursuit and optokinetic gains were reduced, vestibular examinations revealed bilater hyporeflexia. Cranio-corpography and stabilometry showed right vestibulo-spinal deficit with central cervico-cephalic incoordination and pathological body sway even with eyes opened.

Neurotropic (piracetam), neuroactive (citicoline) and vasoactive (pentoxifylline) drugs were employed. A physical and instrumental rehabilitation protocol was planned during 2 weeks of hospitalization. The daily residential program included: VES once a day for 30 min during normal activities; piracetam infusional administration once a day; rehabilitation with a physi-

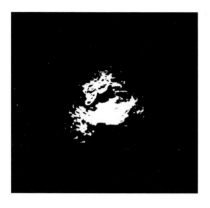 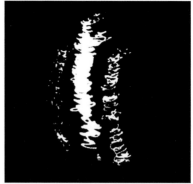

Fig. 4. CCG without collar after 2 weeks   **Fig. 5.** CCG after 3 months

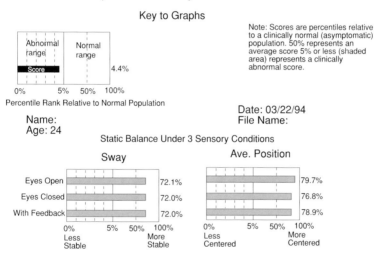

Fig. 6. Stabilometric results after 3 months

otherapist once a day for 1 h, employing VES, 5 days a week; self administered simplest Cawthorne-Cooksey protocol exercises in sitting and supine positions.

The protocol performed with the therapist included:

1. Stepping with eyes opened and closed either on floor or on soft mattress.
2. Postural control with eyes open on soft mattress. When the position is stable, according to the therapist's command the patient must touch, with extended arms and joint hands, with his thumbs some differently coloured targets placed in different positions on a mirror.

3. On the floor looking at himself in a mirror the patient must reach a brick positioned to the back and lateral or front and lateral.
4. "Pointe de mire" exercises maintaining stance on tip toes and/or heels;
5. Balance Master training. Figure 7 shows the limits of stability test. It revealed difficulties in movement time, target sway distance and direction errors especially for right, right-forward and right-backward targets. The training protocol was performed for 30 min once a day every 2 days and it is shown in Fig. 8 with 10 s (A) and 5 s pacings (B).
6. Skitter
   (a) Maintaining correct position under visual feedback control (Fig. 9);
   (b) Visual pointing of targets placed on a mirror (Fig. 10);
   (c) Ankle-hip strategies;
   (d) Oscillations;
   (e) Ankle stability.

PATIENT INFORMATION AND TEST SETTINGS

Patient Name:
Data file:
Target/prot. Type: SP06
Therapy Mode: Beep, Feedback
Post-Test Comment:

Age: 70
Ht.: 171 cm
LOS: 75%

Test Date. 02/16/95
Order #:19
Pacing Speed: 10 sec.

Limits of stability

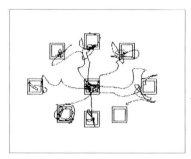

PATH

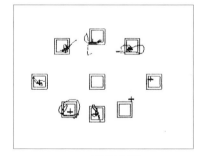

SWAY AREA

Numeric Summary

Transition		Mvt Time (sec)	Path Sway (% Path Len)	Target Sway (% Max Area)	Patient Position (% LOS)	(deg)	Distance Error (% LOS)	Direction Error (deg)
1	(F)	1.48	121.81	0.49	65.9	353.2	-9.1	-6.8
2	(RF)	3.52	236.42	0.76	69.6	45.3	-5.4	0.3
3	(R)	6.84	309.28	N/S	<70.4>	<87.1>	<-4.6>	<-2.9>
4	(RB)	<8.00>	<501.61>	N/A	<61.1>	<116.8>	<-13.9>	<-18.2>
5	(B)	1.90	147.08	0.22	73.9	182.5	-1.1	2.5
6	(LB)	2.56	229.55	0.82	77.3	222.5	2.3	-2.5
7	(L)	4.62	218.26	N/S	<75.2>	<269.2>	<0.2>	<-0.8>
8	(LF)	2.60	204.75	0.13	69.1	317.3	-5.9	2.3

Fig. 7. Limits of stability case n° 2

After 2 weeks, unsteadiness and dizziness were improved subjectively and stabilometry revealed near to normal body sway with eyes closed and normal findings with eyes open and with visual feed-back. The patient continued to perform at home supine, sitting and standing Cawthorne-Cooksey exercises.

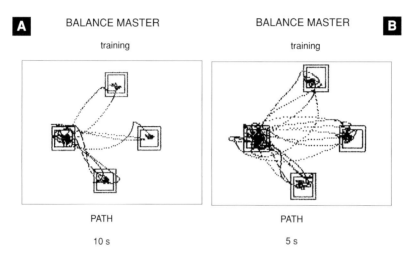

Fig. 8 A, B. Training exercises

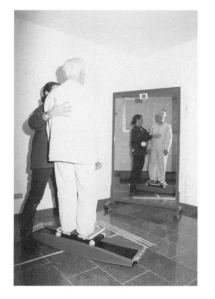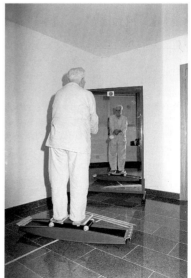

Figs. 9, 10. Skitter exercises under visual feedback control

References

1. Albus JS (1971) A theory of cerebellar function. Mathemathical Biosciences 10:26-61
2. Ashby WR (1956) An introduction to cybernetics. Chapman & Hall Ltd, London
3. Basar E (1980) EEG-brain dynamics. Elsevier, Amsterdam
4. Bertalanffy L von (1962) General system theory. A critical review. General System Yearbook 7:1-20
5. Cherry C (1961) On human communication. Science Ed, New York
6. Cesarani A, Pedotti A, Alpini D (1994) General system theory. A cybernetic basis for modern rehabilitaion treatment of equilibrium disorders. In: Claussen CF, Kirtane MV, Schneider D (eds). Vertigo, nausea, tinnitus and hypoacusia due to central disequilibrium. Edition m+p, Hamburg, p 53
7. Cesarani A, Pedotti A, Alpini A (1994) General system theory. A cybernetic basis for rehabilitative treatment of balance disorders. In: Claussen CF, Kirtane MV, Schneider D (eds). Vertigo, nausea, tinnitus and hypoacusia due to central disequilibrium. Medicin + Pharmacie, Dr Werner Rudat & Co, Nachf, Hamburg
8. Davies PM (1993) Steps to follow. Springer, Heidelberg, Berlin, New York, Tokyo
9. Dilts R, Grinder J, Bandler R, Bandler LC, De Lozier J (1980) Neurolinguistic programming. Meta Publication, Cupertino, California
10. Fujita M (1982) Adapative filter model of the cerebellum. Biological Cybernetics 45:195-206
11. Fujiita M (1982) Simulation of adaptive modification of the vestibulo-ocular reflex with an adaptive filter model of the cerebellum. Biological Cybernetics 45:207-214
12. George FH (1962) The brain as a computer. Pergamon, Oxford
13. Gluck MA, Rumelhart DE (1990) Neuroscience and connectionist theory. Lawrence Erlbaum Associates, Hillsdale, New Jersey
14. Ito M (1982) Cerebellar control of the vestibulo-ocular reflex around the flocculus hypothesis. Annual Rev of Neurosc 5:275-296
15. Ito M (1984) The cerebellum and neural control. New York, Raven
16. Marr D (1969) A theory of cerebellar cortex. J Physiol 202:437-470
17. Mc Culloch WS, Pitts W (1943) A logical calculus of the ideas imminent in nervous activity. Bull Math Biophys 5:115
18. Robinson DA (1976) Adaptive gain control of vestibulo-ocular reflex by the cerebellum. J Neurophys 39(5):954-969
19. Watzlawich P, Beavin JH, Jackson DD (1967) Pragmatic of human communication. W Norton, New York

Subject Index